Energy to Burn

Energy to Burn

The Ultimate Food and Nutrition
Guide to Fuel Your Active Life

JULIE UPTON
and
JENNA BELL-WILSON

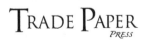

TRADE PAPER PRESS

Trade Paper Press
An imprint of Turner Publishing Company
Nashville, Tennessee
www.turnerpublishing.com

Library of Congress Cataloging-in-Publication Data:

Upton, Julie, date.
  Energy to burn : the ultimate food and nutrition guide to fuel your active life / Julie Upton and Jenna Bell-Wilson.
    p. cm
  Includes bibliographical references and index.
  ISBN 978-0-470-27741-6 (pbk.)
  1. Nutrition. 2. Energy metabolism. I. Bell-Wilson, Jenna A. II. Title.
  RA784.U68   2009
  613—dc22
                                                          2008055981

Printed in the United States of America

10 9 8 7 6 5 4 3 2

This book is dedicated to all the active people
who found their inner athlete as a child
as well as those who awakened it recently.

Contents

Acknowledgments

Energy to Burn wouldn't exist without the aid and support of our very smart colleagues, fit friends, and families. Without their support, it would not have been possible. And thanks to our wonderful spouses, Craig and Willie, whose laid-back personalities are the perfect balances to our high-stress, deadline-driven lives. Without you, we couldn't do what we do.

We would also like to thank our literary agent, John Silbersack, for finding a home for our project and PowerBar and Team Elite for supporting our efforts. We would like to thank our editor, Christel Winkler, for nudging us along (we need to be poked and prodded sometimes) and the entire team at Wiley. You are all superb, and we admire your professionalism and dedication to our book.

Special thanks go out to all the SCAN-registered dietitians, who are a pleasure to work with and are truly the best resources for sound sports nutrition information. Thanks to athlete-dietitian Pamela Nisevich, M.S., R.D., for your help in devising meal plans and menus that fit our guidelines but are also delicious! Thanks to Dana Angelo White, M.S., R.D., ATC/L, for creating specific recipes that taste so great.

I also want to recognize my training partners, who provide endless sports nutrition content and questions while trying to whip me into shape: Bo Arlander, Christine O'Hanlon, Sheila Roebuck, and John Catts; my past and present coaches (including husband Craig), who cut me slack and allow me to test their patience; and to all of my past and present teammates. You are all the best part of being an athlete.

—Julie Upton

I'd like to extend appreciation to my mainstays, who made writing this book possible, training manageable, and my life enjoyable. There are many who deserve my gratitude, but space constraints allow me to call out only a few: thoughtful Pam Nisevich; training partner and confidant, Mitch Mortenson—whom I adore; Karen Morse, my constant; Courtney and Lauren, my heart; Mom and Dad, my inspiration; and Willie, my ultimate support and biggest fan, for whom I am most grateful.

—Jenna A. Bell-Wilson

1

Nutrition Condition

I have always been a top-level athlete, but was never World
Champion material until I got serious about my nutrition.
>   —Kristin Armstrong, World Champion cyclist and Olympic Gold
>   Medalist, road cycling

Athletes often make the mistake of either taking for granted
that their talent will be enough and not realizing the importance of proper nutrition or becoming fanatical about their
nutrition to a point that it becomes a burden.
>   —Michael Johnson, five-time Olympic gold medalist; nine-time
>   world champion in the 200-, 400-, and 4 × 400-meter relay,
>   dubbed "world's fastest man"

Sooner or later athletes realize it's not how hard you train, it's
about how you adapt to training, and that largely depends on
nutrition.
>   —Jeremiah Bishop, professional mountain biker

WE ALL KNOW THE SAYING "YOU ARE WHAT YOU EAT." IT'S NOT ENTIRELY
correct, but we do know that what you eat can make you a better athlete.

We wrote this book to provide readers with the most current, science-
based sports nutrition information and tools to help you eat and drink for
optimal performance. As registered dietitians certified in sports dietetics,
we hear and see firsthand how much sports nutrition misinformation
there is on the Internet, in magazines, and being touted by athletes and
coaches themselves. After talking to hundreds of athletes—from weekend
warriors to world champs—we knew that many athletes would benefit
from a book like this.

Success in sports is determined primarily by your genetic potential and training. However, the most genetically gifted athletes may not be the best because they may have poor conditioning, while athletes with less natural talent—but with good training—may become the world's best in their sport. When you get the combination of great genes and top training, you get a sports phenom. Think of Roger Federer, Tiger Woods, Michael Jordan, and Lance Armstrong. All are genetically gifted and have or had some of the most dedicated training programs of athletes ever in their respective sports.

WHERE DO YOU GET YOUR NUTRITION INFORMATION?

According to a 2008 survey commissioned by the American Dietetic Association, Americans said that their main sources for nutrition information included:

63% TV

45% magazines

24% Internet

19% newspapers

Energy-to-burn nutritionism: Eighty percent of individuals surfing the Web for nutrition information used .com sites and only 20 percent were logging onto more unbiased .gov or .org sites, according to the 2005 survey.

Most athletes never come close to reaching their true potential because their training is suboptimal due to fatigue, recurring injuries, or lack of time, commitment, or motivation. That's where optimal sports nutrition can help. Sports nutrition strategies that provide the right amount of energy and nutrients to facilitate training, recovery, and in-competition fueling can help make up the difference between winning and losing.

Chances are that you probably have your training program under control, probably even have a coach you work with individually or with a team. However, we find that most athletes don't have a "nutrition coach" or hire a sports dietitian for consulting. And, unfortunately, there aren't very many people who are truly qualified to provide evidence-based sports nutrition information. All too often, athletes tell us, "My coach recommended it," or "I know my competition is on this," or "I read about it in a magazine."

Sports Nutrition through the Ages

Ancient Practices

The earliest glimpse into the history of sports nutrition can be found through a historical look at the Olympic Games. Recorded writings from several of these ancient Games provided details about what competitive athletes ate during a typical day and when in competition. While much of this may be more mythical and less factual, records from the 776 B.C. Games are available in sports nutrition textbooks and show that the competitors often consumed gluttonous quantities of animal meats and not much else. Legend has it that Milo of Croton, a wrestler, ate a diet that consisted of twenty pounds of meat, twenty pounds of bread, and eighteen pints of wine a day—a food feat that even Joey Chestnut, the 2007 hot-dog-eating world champion, would have a hard time digesting.

From the ancient Olympic Games until now, virtually every type of diet and nutritional scheme and regimen has been experimented with to enhance athletic performance.

Reports from several subsequent Olympics showed a progression of modern-day thinking about training and nutrition. At the 1936 Olympic Games in Berlin, there was a dramatic shift to recognizing the importance of carbohydrates. While many athletes were still eating a steak, egg, and more steak diet, the Italians, Asians, and Americans were loading up on more grain-based foods such as pasta, rice, and cereal.

Modern Sports Nutrition

Sports nutrition is defined as using eating strategies to promote overall health and wellness, adaptation to training, recovery after training, and optimal performance. The modern science behind the current sports nutrition guidelines is relatively new, with most of the research beginning in the late 1970s, and with most of the major advances in the past two decades.

Much of the sports nutrition research that was originally conducted was on endurance athletes such as marathon runners and cyclists. This is largely because endurance athletes are more likely to become carbohydrate-depleted than athletes in stop-and-go, power-oriented sports, and because endurance athletes need strategies in place to combat the environmental conditions they must compete in for hours on end.

More recently, however, studies have been completed on both team- and power-oriented athletes such as basketball players, baseball players, weight lifters, and skiers. These studies have resulted in new fueling strategies for optimizing the training of strength and power athletes.

Today there are sports nutrition studies on virtually all types of athletes, including race car drivers and pit crews, golfers, sailors, skiers, and snowboarders. Even professional poker players trying to promote their training use nutrition strategies that help keep them at the top of their (card) game.

Whether you're interested in sports nutrition because of an upcoming 5K, century ride, marathon, Ironman competition, or backcountry ski trip, you probably wouldn't expect to be your best physically without breaking a sweat beforehand. Most athletes get the principle of training, and are capable of spending countless hours running or on the bike, in the

GOLD-MEDAL EATS: FUELING OLYMPIANS

The dining area of the Athlete Village for the Summer Games often exceeded the size of three American football fields. In it, the 25,000 Olympians had access to food 24/7 during the three-week Summer Games.

In recent Olympics, athletes have generally been loading up on carbohydrates. According to Michael Crane, the executive chef of the Athens Olympic Games, the most requested food on the 1,500-item World Menu from ARAMARK, the food-service operator for the Games, was rice. Olympians ate more than 250,000 servings of rice during the 2004 Games. Pasta, breads, cereals, and other carbohydrate-rich foods are also mainstays in the diets of Olympians.

It takes more than two thousand cooks and kitchen staff to provide more than two million meals. According to ARAMARK, following are some of the 2004 Olympic food facts:

1,500 menu items

300 tons of produce
  80 different options for fresh fruit
  700,000 apples (the most popular fruit)
  630,000 bananas
  555,000 oranges
  177,000 pounds of potatoes
  nearly 628,000 bananas
  more than 555,000 oranges
  55,800 pints of strawberries
  more than 68,000 pounds of carrots
  nearly 57,000 pounds of onions
  more than 11,000 pounds of mushrooms
  more than 799,000 olives

120 tons of meat
  184,000 pounds of chicken
  119,000 pounds of beef
  72,000 pounds of lamb
  108,000 pounds of pork
20 tons of eggs
225,000 pounds of seafood
3,000 gallons of olive oil
52,000 pounds of cheese
25,000 loaves of bread
more than 20,000 pounds of dry rice
more than 6.6 million servings of water (enough to fill an Olympic-size pool)
2 million cups of coffee
1 million glasses of milk

pool, or in the gym. But what is often overlooked is their nutrition conditioning. Just like you have to strength-train to build muscle, you need to flex your nutrition muscles to optimize your genetic potential and to make the best use of the time you spend training.

PowerBar Athletes and the 2008 Beijing Summer Games

Congratulations to the PowerBar-sponsored athletes who took home an impressive eighteen Olympic medals at the 2008 Summer Games. That's enough medals to put them sixteenth in country medal standings! The medals were won in a variety of sports, including swimming, track and field, rowing, and water polo. Of course, Michael Phelps's record-breaking eight-for-eight gold medals in China add to the PowerBar's longstanding Olympic legacy.

Nutrition Condition Workbook: Find Your Energy Quotient (EQ)

Think of the nutrition basics like strengthening your core; it's essential for just about any type of physical demand you're going to place on your body.

Throughout the book, we build upon your nutrition foundation with more sports-specific nutrition tools such as pre-event meals, nutritional periodization, recovery nutrition, fluid and hydration guidelines, supplements, and a fourteen-day energy-to-burn eating plan with recipes and tips for maximum energy. But first let's make sure you have the foundation of healthy eating mastered before we amp it up.

A healthy diet can be achieved with a few important, albeit somewhat vague, concepts: adequacy, variety, balance, moderation, and nutrient density. We'll explain all of this nutritionese below. But first, take our Energy Quotient (EQ) quiz to see how well you're doing right now.

How's Your EQ (or Nutrition Condition)?

To determine your EQ, read the statements in the following sections to see if you agree or disagree with them. If you agree with them mostly, your EQ is on track. If your eating patterns are in stark contrast to the statements within each section, you'll be happy to know that by following the principles in this book, you should be able to eke much more out of your training and in competition.

Nutrition Condition Principle I: Variety

1. I really try to make my meals different most days of the week.
2. I try to include colorful foods in most of my meals and snacks.
3. I'm an adventurous eater; I will try just about anything, and I don't restrict myself from eating anything.
4. I like to add vegetables to my sandwich, fruit to my snacks, and create a dish with a variety of ingredients.
5. The bulk of my diet comes from whole foods such as fruits, vegetables and whole grains, and I try to eat fewer overly processed foods.
6. I am an equal opportunity eater—I eat from a variety of food groups every day.
7. I can recite the five major food groups from the USDA Pyramid.
8. I like more than pasta and bagels. I also eat white and brown rice, quinoa, bulger, popcorn, and other grains.
9. When I travel for events, I love trying the cuisine of the regions.
10. I try to think of the seasonality of what I eat, and whenever possible, I try to include the freshest ingredients in my meals.

You know the saying "Variety is the spice of life," and there's no better way to ensure that you're getting all the vitamins, minerals, and other bioactive compounds foods provide without eating a wide variety of foods most days. There are at least forty different essential nutrients that you need daily just to prevent malnutrition, and most likely many more to optimize athletic performance. There is no single food or category of foods that can provide us with all the nutrients we need. Eating a wide variety of foods will make sure that you have the right nutrients for growth, metabolic processes, and the energy you need to fuel your activities, but not so much that you gain excess body fat.

Not only does eating a variety of foods ensure that you get the nutrients you need, it also protects you from getting too much of a specific nutrient. Even water is toxic if you drink too much of it! Foods are made up of complex bioactive compounds such as vitamins and minerals. When we eat foods, these compounds act synergistically with other foods and nutrients. That's why by ingesting a vitamin and mineral supplement, you cannot expect the same health benefits as from eating a food that is rich in those nutrients. This is also why many studies with isolated compounds from foods such as beta-carotene and vitamins C and E show little benefit for reducing the risk of disease, and sometimes these nutrients, given on their own, have been shown to increase the risk for certain diseases.

To help you get the most out of your food choices, refer to the fourteen-day energy-to-burn eating plan and shopping list. If you follow these recommendations, you will basically guarantee that you're getting enough variety in your diet.

Nutrition Condition Principle II: Energy Balance

1. I feel like I have enough energy to do things I want to do on most if not all days of the week.
2. I strive to consume enough energy-rich foods to sustain my workout.
3. I try to let hunger be my guide as to when and how much I eat.
4. I adjust my energy intake during the off-season.
5. I avoid "fad diets."
6. My weight is fairly consistent and only varies by about five to ten pounds from when I'm training to the off-season.
7. I understand the difference between hunger and appetite.
8. I make a conscious effort not to reach for food to help alleviate boredom, stress, or when I'm feeling down.
9. Coffee or other sources of caffeine are part of my daily life, but I don't rely on them to get me through the day.
10. I try to eat frequently—every three or so hours—so that I never feel totally ravenous.

As an athlete, you need energy to be your best, but it's a fine balance between having enough energy to fuel your activities but not too much to fuel fat stores. Finding the right energy balance isn't always easy. It comes naturally for many athletes, but for others, who may have a real love of food, be more emotional eaters, or have naturally higher body fat compositions, it's much harder to balance their intake with exercise. In sports where thinness is less important, energy balance is less important, but for endurance athletes, gymnasts, and most master athletes, finding balance between how much and what you eat and exercise is critical.

We have found that optimal energy balance to promote a lean body mass is one of the best ways to go from a mere chump to a champ. Three-time Hawaii Ironman champion Peter Reid explained that it wasn't until he lost 10 pounds in the off-season that he started to win Ironman distance events. The same is true for pro mountain biker Jeremy Horgan-Kobelski, who also dropped 10 pounds and then went on to win the national championship. One of the most dramatic transformations we've seen is by Cody Wilson, who lost more than 120 pounds and became one of the best BMXers in the world. Numerous amateur and professional athletes have told us that they basically experienced breakthroughs after they learned how to better balance their energy input and output.

To help, in the past few years, sports nutritionists have introduced the idea of nutrition periodization, a strategy for designing meal plans and energy and macronutrient distribution patterns to closely match energy and nutritional needs to the demands of training and competition. In a practical sense, it means that during the course of a year, a month, or a week, your diet may change to be higher or lower in calories, proteins, and carbohydrates to help maintain energy balance and optimize the performance goal, like recovery versus high-intensity training.

This book provides several chapters that deal with how to match your nutrition to your exercise and body composition goals. We have strategies for endurance athletes in peak training versus strategies for bodybuilders seeking gains in muscle mass. We have a chapter for dealing with how to find your best body weight and how to get there (and stay there!).

Nutrition Condition Principle III: Moderation

1. When I use butter, mayonnaise, or a high-fat condiment, I try to stick with small servings.
2. I avoid overconsuming any single food to the point where I feel stuffed or sick of it.
3. When having a dessert, I'll enjoy a small piece of candy or chocolate or a cookie or two, rather than an entire bag or box.
4. I avoid "super-size" portions of "junk" foods such as candy, sodas, or other high-fat desserts.
5. I understand the nutrition labels on food packages and often look at them when I'm shopping.
6. I am aware of unhealthy saturated and trans fats, and know where they lurk.
7. Having a celebratory drink is part of my reward for training, but I try not to overdo alcohol.
8. I try not to fixate on my diet every day, and I just try to make sure it balances out over the week.

9. When it comes to beverages, I really don't supersize any drinks.

10. I like to snack, but I try not to make snacking my fourth or fifth meal.

Of the three nutrition pillars—balance, variety, and moderation—moderation is the most vague and hard to define. When we tell people to eat in moderation, it is always up to debate and one's personal interpretation. And when we talk about foods to have in moderation, it's because they're loaded with "negative" nutrients. The main negative nutrients in the U.S. diet are saturated fat, trans fats, cholesterol, added sugars, and sodium. We also include alcohol because it's addictive and too much is not a good thing.

We define moderation with athletes as having the appropriate number of servings of foods and beverages to promote optimal training, competition, and recovery. When you let your portions get overboard your diet becomes disproportionate, and you're not practicing moderation. Moderation isn't just about restricting serving sizes; it is also about allowing you to have foods that may be more caloric than they are nutritionally worth in moderation.

Fortunately, we'll be providing more details about food sources of the negative nutrients that athletes need to be concerned about, and details about what exactly you should be eating more of and those items you need to eat less of. Practicing moderation also is a way to temper overall intake so that one food or beverage doesn't become the focus of the diet—however nutritious it may be. More simply, "Enough is good; more isn't always better."

Now that you've determined your EQ, let's look at the nutrition basics covered by the new Dietary Guidelines.

MyPyramid Anatomy: What Uncle Sam Says You Should Eat

Every five years, we have the Olympics in the nutrition world. This is when the government releases the new dietary guidance systems that affect our entire food supply as well as what our kids eat at school, what farmers will get paid to farm, and the images that food manufacturers put all over their packages.

The last Nutrition Olympics were in 2005, when the U.S. Department of Agriculture (USDA) along with the Department of Health and Human

Services (DHHS) released the dietary guidelines for Americans to tell us what and how much we should eat to live longer and healthier lives.

The dietary guidelines are based on the scientific evidence about food and all the macro- and micronutrients, and their relations to chronic diseases, especially heart disease, diabetes, cancer, and obesity. Since more than two-thirds of the U.S. adult population is either overweight or obese, there is much emphasis on balancing calories with exercise to help achieve an ideal body weight.

The dietary guidelines are not meant to treat or cure an illness, nor are they designed for people with special nutritional concerns. As an athlete, you fall into that special nutritional concern category, so we'll help you adapt what's appropriate from the dietary guidelines to assist you in attaining your goals.

The new dietary guidelines provide several key recommendations for healthy individuals. A review of these major guidelines is shown below, along with a sample menu of what a diet would look like that followed the new guidelines.

Eat Nutrient-Packed Foods

Eat nutrient-dense foods and beverages within and among the basic food groups while limiting those foods and beverages that deliver little nutrition (basically, get the junk out).

Athlete Adaptation: Eat the majority of your diet from the five food groups. The specific sports nutrition products (bars, gels, drinks) fit technically into your discretionary calories according to the government. Since you exercise, you have much more leeway to get the carbohydrate-rich sports nutrition products to enhance performance.

Watch Your Weight

Balance your food intake with your activity level to keep your weight stable over time.

Athlete Adaptation: Unless you're a sumo wrestler or an offensive lineman, added body fat does little to improve athletic performance. We don't care as much about your weight on a scale, but we will help you manage your energy intake so that you maximize leanness.

Get Physical

Strive for sixty to ninety minutes a day of physical activity, including cardio, strength training, and stretching.

Athlete Adaptation: Since you bought this book, you probably are already meeting or exceeding this target. (The government's guidelines count all movement, from walking the dog to gardening, as physical activity.)

Eat More Fruits and Vegetables, Whole Grains, and Dairy Products

Eat a variety of colorful fruits and vegetables. Strive for at least 2 cups of fruit and 2½ cups of vegetables per day. Eat 3 or more servings of whole grains each day. Consume three servings of nonfat or low-fat dairy products daily.

Athlete Adaptation: It's what Mom always said: "Eat your fruits and vegetables." Produce and whole grains are loaded with key vitamins, minerals, and phytochemicals that may help with recovery. Three servings a day of dairy products or dairy alternatives are advised because they pack in calcium, vitamin D, potassium, and many other nutrients that most of us lack.

Carbohydrate Choices

Choose fiber-rich fruits, vegetables, and whole grains as your main sources of carbohydrates. Choose and prepare foods with little added sugars or caloric sweeteners.

Athlete Adaptation: Carbohydrates are the muscles' preferred fuel source, and your brain and nervous system can only utilize blood glucose for energy. The vast majority of an athlete's daily calories—up to 65 percent—should come from carbohydrates. Generally, we aim for 2.3 to 4.5 grams carbohydrate/pound of body weight for your daily diet (equal to 5 to 10 grams CHO/kilogram of body weight). For a 150-pound athlete, carbohydrates would total 345 to 675 grams of carbohydrates per day, depending on the type of training and performance goals.

Mind Your Fats

Eat less than 10 percent of calories from saturated fat, and less than 300 milligrams per day of dietary cholesterol, and keep trans fats as low as possible. Keep total fat between 20 and 35 percent of total calories.

Athlete Adaptation: The dietary fat intakes of athletes vary greatly from sport to sport. Endurance athletes often consume 27 to 35 percent of their calories as fat, while athletes in sports such as gymnastics and figure skating often consume lower amounts of fat. Research shows that there are no performance benefits from adhering to a diet with less than 15 percent of calories from fat.

As long as the source of fat is healthy (this will be discussed later), you can consume up to 40 percent of total calories from fat without any adverse effects. Many endurance athletes find that a more generous fat intake is the only way that they can reach their daily calorie goals. Conversely, for athletes who need to lose weight, fat is reduced to keep protein and carbohydrate sufficient to fuel exercise while losing weight. In general, athletes can strive to have .45 gram fat per pound of body weight (1 gram of fat/kilogram of body weight).

Sodium and Potassium Pointers

Consume less than a teaspoon of salt per day and limit processed foods rich in sodium and include plenty of potassium-rich foods, such as fresh produce.

Athlete Adaptation: Sodium is generally not a concern for individuals who are active. In fact, too little sodium for those who are sweating poses more health risk than too much sodium. Athletes can easily enjoy foods that contain liberal amounts of sodium, such as snack chips and pretzels as well as processed foods, without worry.

Drink Alcohol in Moderation

Responsible, healthful drinking equals up to one drink for women, two for men. A "drink" equals 12 ounces of beer, 6 ounces of wine, or 1½ ounces of distilled spirits.

Athlete Adaptation: You can rehydrate with alcoholic beverages (we don't recommend it), but it's untrue that beer is rich in carbohydrates and can be used either to carbohydrate-load or to speed recovery. Athletes can enjoy alcohol in moderation, and we find that most athletes do enjoy wine, beer, or spirits as part of their diets. Many feel that a drink is their treat for accomplishing a hard training day or competition.

MyPyramid

You may wonder what the MyPyramid has to do with the dietary guidelines. Well, consider the Pyramid (accessed at www.MyPyramid.gov) Cliffs Notes, or *Dietary Guidelines for Dummies*. Basically, the MyPyramid takes all the dietary guidelines and condenses them into one visual.

At www.MyPyramid.gov you can enter your sex, age, and activity level and get one of twelve semi-personalized versions. This is fine for most female athletes, but for males who exercise more than two hours a day, the MyPyramid may not provide enough calories to fulfill your energy needs. The new MyPyramid is in 3D, with vertical multicolor bands representing each of the food groups. Here's what the colors stand for:

orange = grains

green = vegetables

red = fruit

yellow = oils

blue = dairy or dairy alternatives

purple = lean meat, fish, and meal alternatives

The depiction of a person climbing up the pyramid signifies that physical activity is as important as what you eat.

Athlete Adaptation: As an athlete, your daily servings of foods will change based on your training and athletic goals. The number of calories and macronutrient distribution needs to adapt as you train less or more, lose or gain weight, or are competing.

And depending on the time of year, your diet may contain much more fat than what the Pyramid recommends, especially if you are an endurance athlete in heavy training. Similarly, athletes needing to build muscle or seeking strength gains will need more protein servings than the government allots daily.

2,000-Calorie Sample from USDA MyPyramid

This calorie level recommends the following number of servings from each food group. A 2,000-calorie diet is the standard diet by which all food labels provide a percentage of Recommended Daily Value.

Grains	6 ounces
Vegetables	2.5 cups
Fruits	2 cups
Milk	3 cups
Lean meats	5.5 ounces
Oils	6 teaspoons

2,600-Calorie Sample from USDA MyPyramid

Here are the number of servings from each of the six food groups for a 2,600-calorie diet:

Grains	9 ounces
Vegetables	3.5 cups
Fruits	2 cups
Milk	3 cups
Lean meats	6.5 ounces
Oils	8 teaspoons

WHAT'S A SERVING?

While we don't necessarily use the USDA serving sizes, it is good to know what they are, because they're probably much skimpier than what you consider a serving. Also, to confuse you even more, the USDA servings are often different from the servings you'll see on a food package. We have outlined many typical athlete meal plans in chapters 10 and 11 as part of our Eating for Energy suggested meals and snack combinations.

Grains and Whole Grains
- ½ cup cooked rice, pasta, or cooked cereal
- 1 ounce dry pasta or rice
- 1 slice bread
- 1 cup flaked cereal

Vegetables
- 2 cups leafy greens
- 1 cup chopped or cooked vegetable
- 1 cup juice

Fruits
- 1 cup raw fruit
- 1 cup 100% fruit juice
- 1 large banana or peach
- 1 small apple
- 1 medium pear
- 8 strawberries
- ½ cup blueberries, blackberries

Milk, Dairy, and Dairy Substitutes
- 1 cup milk or yogurt
- 1½ ounces natural cheese
- 2 ounces processed cheese

Meat & Beans
- 1 ounce lean meat, fish, poultry
- 1 egg
- ½ cup cooked dry beans or tofu
- 1 tbsp peanut butter or other nut butter
- ½ ounce nuts or seeds

Fats & Oils
- 1 tsp vegetables oil or trans-fat–free soft margarine
- 1 tsp mayonnaise
- 8 large olives
- ⅓ ounce most nuts
- ¾ tsp peanut butter

Here's what a 2,600-calorie Uncle Sam diet would look like:

Breakfast
1½ cups whole grain flaked cereal (3 whole grain)
1 cup skim or 1% milk (1 milk)
1 8-ounce glass orange juice (1 fruit)
Coffee or tea

Snack
1 small apple (1 cup fruit)
Pria French Vanilla Crisp Bar (170 calories)

Lunch
Turkey sandwich
   2 slices whole-grain bread (2 whole grain)
   2 ounces turkey breast (2 ounces meat)
   1 ounce slice provolone cheese (1 ounce)
   lettuce, tomato (1 vegetable)
   2 tsp mayonnaise (2 fat)
Side salad
   2 cups salad greens (1 vegetable)
   1 cup mixed, chopped vegetables (1 vegetable)
   ⅓ cup shredded cheese (1 milk)
   2 tbsp Italian salad dressing (2 fat)

Dinner
3½ ounces broiled chicken breast (3½ ounces meat)
1 cup cooked broccoli (1 vegetable)
2 tsp olive oil (2 fat)
2 ounce dinner roll (2 grain)
1½ tsp butter (50 discretionary calories)
Dessert: 1 cup frozen nonfat yogurt (1 milk)

Snack
1 12-ounce light beer (110 discretionary calories)
2 ounces pretzels (2 grain)

NUTRIENT DENSITY: FINDING THE HARD-WORKING CALORIES

Nutrient density may arguably be the most helpful concept to consider when you're about to bite into something. It refers to the amount of nutrition a food contains in relation to its calorie value. If it is nutrient-dense, it is rich in vitamins, minerals, phytochemicals, fiber, and other good stuff, without being loaded with calories. It's more bang for your buck. You want harder-working calories in your diet, not freeloading calories.

Foods that have a low nutrient density, such as soft drinks, candy, and sugar, are often referred to as "empty calories." Not surprisingly, the most nutrient-dense foods are fruits, vegetables, 100 percent fruit and vegetable juices, low-fat dairy foods, and lean meat. These nutritional all-stars supply many different nutrients and phytochemicals with few calories. Just think how many people have blamed their weight gain on their obsession with leafy greens or brussels sprouts. Plus, there's something researchers have found about nutrient-dense foods: they help keep us fuller longer, so you're less likely to overeat. By choosing nutrient-dense foods, you are making your calories work for you, not against you!

In the future, there may be a standard for food packages to help you identify the foods that are most nutrient-dense within their category. So within the breads, cereals, and grains food group, the foods that provide the most nutrients per calories would be easily identified. A few other countries have adopted strategies to help individuals make wiser food choices. Until these food scores are made available, the best bet is to read the nutrition facts panel and ingredients list to know what you're buying. Research shows that label readers have healthier diets than those who skip the nutrition facts panel on packages.

Putting It All Together for Performance

There is no special food or "cocktail" combination of nutrients we can prescribe that will miraculously improve your performance, but your biggest boost can be realized if you follow an eating plan that is balanced and provides a variety of nutrient-rich foods.

Throughout this book you will read chapters that will help you achieve an optimal diet for energy. You'll learn what's best for pre-, during, and post-competition as well as proper hydration, recovery, ways to achieve a leaner body, and which vitamins, minerals, or supplements will boost performance.

2

Your Perfect Weight: How to Find It and Keep It

I lost ten pounds during the off-season, got stronger, and started winning.
—*Peter Reid, three-time Ironman world champion*

I'm motivated to eat better because I want to keep my weight down for climbing . . . and for appearances.
—*Ariel Jakobovits, road cyclist*

ATHLETES COME IN ALL SHAPES AND SIZES. IT'S MOST APPARENT WHEN YOU compare the heights and weights of the world's best athletes in their respective sports. There are laws of physics that largely determine why NFL and NBA players are huge, top runners are small, and distance swimmers have more body fat than other endurance athletes.

When looking at the bios of the world's best athletes, it's common to see 150-pound differences in weight and more than 1-foot difference in height between average athlete size. There are exercise physiologists who study the body size and composition of athletes and who have developed formulas to predict who will be better at a particular sport just based on anthropometric information. What's even more striking is watching athletes who cross over from one sport to another and how the body morphs with the demands of their new sport.

Brawny Man to Scrawny Man

Julie's husband, Craig, who was on the New Zealand national water polo team for years, while playing water polo weighed 210 pounds for his 6-foot,

3-inch frame. He recalls having less than 10 percent body fat at the time. After many successful years in the pool, he then decided to become a pro cyclist. After initial success in New Zealand and Australia, he was picked up by an Italian team to race in Europe. To be competitive in the European pro peloton, where the climbs are longer and steeper than Down Under, Craig had to be lighter. In one season, he lost 55 pounds. Since he's remained a road cyclist for more than a decade, he's maintained about 160 to 165 pounds. Since few cyclists are over 6 feet tall, and there are advantages of being smaller and lighter in road cycling, Craig is always conscious of his weight to help compensate for his height.

> Tour de France climbers generally weigh about 2 pounds per inch. For a 6-foot athlete, that's a feathery 144 pounds.

Clearly, there are biomechanical advantages for specific body sizes and types for sports. Your weight and body composition are two key factors that affect exercise performance. Body weight and composition affect speed, endurance, power, strength, and agility. While you cannot change how tall you are, or your age, sex, or parents, all these play a role in your body composition. However, as with most athletes, proper training and an appropriate diet and fueling strategy can help you achieve an ideal body composition.

While there are always the exceptions to the norms, body size affects performance. Swimmers with long limbs need fewer strokes to propel themselves across the pool. Runners need to be light and have slim legs because they need to lift their legs off the ground to propel themselves thousands of times during each run. On the other hand, football or basketball players need more mass and power to be able to move the weight of opposing athletes. Triathletes, as well as other multisport athletes, tend to have varying body sizes because they need to excel at a variety of disciplines.

Unless you're a sumo wrestler or lineman or you are planning to swim the English Channel, a leaner frame will improve your performance. On the contrary, friends who have trained for the English Channel, trans Tahoe, and other swims have benefited from packing on extra body fat as insulation for the cold-water environments. In fact, recently a friend attempted to swim trans Tahoe solo, but he couldn't finish due to hypothermia. At about 6 to 7 percent body fat, it would naturally be hard for him to make the 11.5-mile crossing in water temps in the high fifties. However, put him in the Hawaii Ironman and he excels in the bike and run. For the majority of sports, leanness doesn't guarantee fitness, but following a performance-oriented eating plan and solid training should help you get to your ideal body composition.

We know this isn't a diet book, and to us, *diet* is a four-letter word. However, optimal body weight and leanness are, by far, the top concerns of athletes—men and women alike and in a wide variety of sports. That's because most athletes understand that body fat is like deadweight, or weight that cannot help propel or accelerate the body whether you need to run, jump, twist, or throw.

Advantages of Fat Loss

Surprisingly, there is little published research on the performance outcomes of reducing body fat or body weight among athletes. This is often because as a group, elite athletes (the athletes whom most researchers study) are already generally very lean, so there is not enough differentiation in body fat among them to assess performance outcomes in relation to body fat. In addition, in sports where athletes have to reach weight limits, such as boxing and wrestling, attaining a certain weight decides whether one can compete. Despite the lack of published studies on the benefits of reducing body fat percentages among athletes, we have heard from hundreds of athletes who aren't shy about telling us how much better they perform after losing excess body fat.

One study showed that when runners had extra weight, their performance decreased by 30 percent. For sports where there is a subjective, aesthetic component, such as gymnastics and diving, there are no data to support the theory that leanness improves performance. However, it is thought that judges of these sports have inherent biases toward athletes with leaner physiques.

Based on studies, a distance runner runs 2 seconds faster per mile for every 1 pound lost. And for every 5 pounds lost, a cyclist rides 1.5 seconds faster for a 4,000-meter race and 15 seconds faster over a 40-kilometer time trial.

According to Performance Labs HC, a cycling and multisport training facility, here are the watts per kilogram that correspond with road cycling categories and how impactful weight loss can be for improving the power-to-weight ratio.

Cat V male = 2.8 watts/kg

Cat IV male = 3.5 watts/kg (female 2.8 w/kg)

Cat III male = 4 watts/kg (female 3.2 w/kg)

Cat II male = 4.3 watts/kg (female 3.6 w/kg)

Cat 1 male = 4.7 watts/kg (female 4 w/kg)

World Class male and female athlete >5 watts/kg

Tour de France winner: 6.5 to 7 watts/kg

Based on these estimates, losing 15 to 20 pounds for a male or 10 to 15 pounds for a female would move each up a category.

Finding Your Body Composition: Are You Overfat or Underlean?

Since body weight on a regular scale tells us how much we weigh, including fat, muscle, bone, and water, it does nothing to indicate if we're carrying excess weight. That's why the scale is okay if it's used in conjunction with some other way to tell how much of that weight is muscle versus fat.

Looking at body weight alone, you can mistakenly believe that some athletes are fitter than others. For example, two athletes of equal height and weight may have surprisingly different body compositions. If a woman who weighs 120 pounds has 25 percent body fat (30 pounds of fat), she's "fatter" than a woman who weighs 135 pounds who has 20 percent body fat (27 pounds of fat).

Body composition differs from person to person and athlete to athlete, and is highly individualized based on sex, race, genetics, and other factors. Unfortunately, there are no standards that suggest what optimal percentage body fat levels are for athletes of various sports.

From several research studies that have collected body fat percentages of elite athletes (including professionals and Olympians), some average percentages for various sports have emerged. Keep in mind, though, that it is hard to interpret this information, since some studies may have used underwater weighing and others skinfold calipers or bioelectric impedance to assess body composition.

Sport	Percent Body Fat Male	Percent Body Fat Female
Marathoners	3–5	15
Ironman competitors	5–11	7–17
Swimmers	6–7	18
Basketball	9–10	23
Gymnastics	6	17
Ice hockey	9	—

Sport	Percent Body Fat Male	Percent Body Fat Female
Football, linemen	17–18	—
Alpine skiers	12	20
Cross-country skiers	10	18
Tennis	11	22
Bodybuilders	9	13
Road cyclists	11	15
Baseball/softball	13	19
Sprinters	16.5	19
Discus/shot put	16–18	25–28
Wrestlers	8	—
Sumo wrestlers	27	—
Speed skaters	7	16–17
Volleyball	10	18
Minimum for health	3–5	12
Acceptable for health	10–15	20–25

Tools to Test if You Are Overly Fat or Underweight

Sports dietitians have many ways to assess body fat, but also there are several ways to gauge how lean you are on your own.

BMI Calculator

You may remember the old height and weight tables, which have pretty much fallen by the wayside. Now, the new gold standard used by public health officials is the body mass index (BMI calculator).

The body mass index is correlated to body fat in most normal-weight individuals but is not the best for extremely fit athletes. However, because it does not directly measure fat mass or lean mass, it is not as sensitive as other body fat measuring tools, such as bioelectric impedance, skinfold measures, or underwater weighing. In addition, the BMI has no indication of where the fat is. Is it subcutaneous, visceral, or primarily in the thighs and butt? As an athlete, you can use the BMI as a general guide, but don't consider it your best predictor of body composition.

Body mass index can be calculated using pounds and inches:

$$BMI = \frac{\text{weight in pounds} \times 703}{\text{height in inches}^2}$$

For example, a 174.5-pound, 6-foot male has a BMI of 23.6: (174.5 × 703) ÷ 72^2.

BMI	Assessment	Percent Body Fat White	Percent Body Fat African American	Percent Body Fat Asian
<18.5	Underweight	21	20	25
18.5–24.9	Normal	33	32	40
25–29.9	Overweight	NA	NA	NA
30 and above	Obese	39	41	41

Source: CDC and AJCN Dec 11, 2005; www.cdc.gov/NCCDPHP/DNPA/BMI/bmi-adult.htm

Following are some examples of BMI scores for athletes from various sports. As you can see, athletes come in all sizes and shapes. However, despite wide differences in height and weight, virtually all the athletes fall between 18 and 25, which is considered normal or healthy. You will find endurance athletes at the lower end of normal and ball sport athletes at the higher end. Use this as a guide when evaluating your BMI and your body.

Athlete	Height/Weight	BMI
Landon Donovan, USA Soccer	5' 8"/148	22.5
Lance Armstrong, USA Cycling	5' 10"/158	22.7
Levi Leipheimer, USA Cycling	5' 7"/136	21.3
Shaquille O'Neal, NBA	7' 1"/325	31.6
Tom Brady, NFL	6' 4"/225	27.4
Deena Kastor, USA Track and Field	5' 4"/104	17.8
Meb Keflezighi USA Track and Field	5' 7"/127	19.9
Dan Browne, USA Track and Field	5' 9"/145	21.4
Jen Rhines, USA Track and Field	5' 3"/105	18.6
Michael Phelps, USA Swimming	6' 4"/195	23.7
Katie Smith, WNBA	5'11"/174	24.3
Derek Jeter, MLB	6' 3"/195	24.4
Tiger Woods, PGA	6' 1"/185	24.4
Hunter Kemper, USA Triathlon	6' 3"/167	20.9
Serena Williams, USTA	5' 9"/139	20.5
Kristin Armstrong, USA Cycling	5' 6"/126	20.3

Waist Circumference

Waist measurements are becoming the new best predictor of risk for developing heart disease and diabetes. The waist measurement is indirectly assessing the amount of visceral or deep belly fat you have. This fat is dangerous because it is most closely linked with high blood pressure, abnormal blood lipids, insulin resistance, and inflammation. In fact, elevated waist circumference is fast becoming one of the best predictors for overall health and well being.

Researchers at St. Luke's Roosevelt Obesity Research Center in New York City and Canadian researchers have reported that waist cutoffs correspond to increased risk for disease. These studies were used among nonathletes, so these values are a general guide.

Waist Circumference	Male	Female
Normal	<35	<31
Overly fat	35–42	31–40
Obese	>43	>41

Waist circumference and not body mass index explains obesity-related health risk. To measure your waist, a tape measure should be snug horizontally around the level of the top of your iliac crest (hip bones), where your waist would be narrowest. Take the measurement as you exhale a normal breath. For men, waist circumference should be less than or equal to 35 inches. Women should strive for a waist circumference of up to 31 inches.

Pounds per Inch

In the 1970s and 1980s, a few formulas were developed to provide a crude calculation of ideal body weight. The Devine formula is one of those. This obviously would not work for power lifters or elite marathoners, but for the average runner, triathlete, swimmer, or ball sport athlete, it's a good place to start. Just don't use this as a gold standard to assess your body composition.

Women: 100 pounds for 5 feet, and 5 pounds for every inch thereafter. A 5-foot, 7-inch woman would have a 135-pound ideal body weight.

Men: 110 pounds for 5 feet, and 5 pounds for every additional inch. A 6-foot man would have a 170-pound ideal body weight.

Pinch and Inch

This is an old standby that may seem unscientific but may have some merit. Using your thumb and index finger, if you can pinch more than an inch of subcutaneous fat in your belly, you're overly fat.

THE EVER-EXPANDING MLB, NFL, AND NBA
BALLPLAYERS: XL TO XXXL

There has been an incredible increase in the heights and weights of high school, collegiate, and professional football, basketball, and baseball players. While some of the increases may be due, in part, to designer drugs, diet also has played a role in the larger-than-life sizes of many pro athletes. The downside to this increased girth is that research suggests that many pro football players are, well, fat.

This is a sign also that you may be apple-shaped, and therefore at increased risk of heart disease and diabetes due to excess abdominal fat, which is known to increase risk for cardiovascular disease, diabetes, and chronic inflammation.

_____ subcutaneous inches in hand (1–1.5 inches is normal; >1.5 inches is high).

Measuring Your Body Composition

As we've said, it's not how much you weigh, it's how much of that weight is fat and muscle that really matters. The only way to really know is to use one of the several techniques that have been developed to measure body composition.

These days, health clubs, sports expos, hospitals, and performance labs across the country offer high-tech ways to get your percentage of body fat calculated. Here is a look at each method and how reliable the results are. In general, we recommend using one of the easier techniques, such as bio-electric impedance or skinfold calipers (with a well-trained technician), because you'll be more likely to get retested. It's not good enough to get tested once; you want to repeat your body composition three to four times per year: preseason, midseason, and postseason. This will help track how your body composition is throughout the year and whether you are getting too lean or not lean enough when it really matters the most.

Hydrodensitometry (Underwater Weighing)

Long considered the gold standard for body composition testing, this technique is based on the fact that fat is less dense than fat-free tissue. It requires submerging the athlete in a tank to measure the water and air displacement. Newer techniques, such as DEXA body scans, are now generally used instead of underwater weighing.

Dual-Energy X-ray Absorptiometry (DEXA) Scans

DEXA is generally available only at research facilities and is the most precise technique to measure body fat. DEXA uses a whole body scanner to detect bone and soft tissue mass. It can take less than ten minutes and is about the most accurate way of testing your true body fat. Bonus: you'll get the health of your bones at the same time. The only downsides are that the test can be expensive and it can be hard to find a facility that has the equipment.

Bioelectric Impedance Analysis (BIA) Scales

These scales have gotten better and less expensive over the years. They use a low-level electrical current to travel through the body to determine the amount of muscle and fat. The fat impedes an electrical current and water; this is an indirect way of measuring muscle mass.

BIA scales are available from Tanita, Homedics, and Health O Meter, all of which have been found to be well correlated to underwater weighing. They have about a 4 percent margin of error. One problem with BIA scales is that hydration status, skin temperature, and food intake impact the readings. It's best to test at the same time of day and when you are adequately hydrated.

Skinfold Calipers

Skinfold caliper readers measure the thickness of the fat layer on specific body sites (arms, thighs, abdomen, chest, and back). The reliability of the results of calipers is dependent on who is taking the measurements and the calibration of the calipers. Use calipers to monitor changes in your body fat over time. It's also important to always use the same technician.

Weight Loss Workbook: Steps to Lose More Fat and Keep More Muscle

If you have successfully assessed your body composition and know that you have some excess body fat to tackle, here we deal with how to lose the fat and keep the muscle.

First, despite what you may have heard, it can be challenging to lose body fat entirely when you lose weight. In fact, for every pound you lose, you will always lose some lean body mass, and that has much to do with how drastically you cut your calories and protein intake and how much body fat you currently have.

However, no matter how slow or how fast you lose weight, some percentage of the weight loss will be nonfat mass. An interesting review of studies showed that you can lose 80 percent nonfat mass when losing weight when you are lean to begin with and attempt to cut calories too drastically. In the best-case scenarios, which have been done with overweight or obese individuals, they can lose a higher percentage of fat mass when they adhere to a diet and exercise program. However, individuals with 10 or 15 percent body fat to start with will lose more than 50 percent fat-free mass when losing weight.

To maximize fat loss, it's important to take the right steps to lose weight, which is to only moderately cut calories and watch nutrient timing and protein quality in the diet to help spare as much lean tissue as possible. Most research suggests that a combination of diet and exercise is best for achieving weight loss and keeping it off. However, when it comes to just losing weight, diet is the most effective. Consider this study: Six endurance-trained men followed a diet with a 1,000-calorie-per-day deficit for seven days by either (a) exercising more while maintaining their caloric intake, or (b) eating less while keeping exercise the same. The exercise group lost only 1.67 pounds, and the diet group lost 4.75 pounds. However, other studies in well-controlled environments have found that whether the caloric deficit is attained by diet or exercise, the net weight loss should be the same.

We recommend a combination of diet and exercise, with an emphasis on diet until you reach your goal body composition.

Step One: Calculate Your Calorie Needs

The first step to losing weight is to determine how many calories you currently eat to sustain your weight. Then, from there, we reduce those calories by 500 to 1,000 calories a day through a combination of diet changes and exercise to promote weight loss.

Use the following calculation to determine your calorie need; then multiply it by the activity factor to determine your overall calorie requirements to lose weight. Start by calculating your resting metabolic rate (RMR). (To convert your height from inches to centimeters, multiply by 2.54. To convert your weight in pounds to kilograms, divide by 2.2.)

Harris Benedict Equation for Resting Metabolic Rate (RMR)

Men: RMR = 88.36 + (4.8 × ht. in cm) + (13.4 × wt. in kg)
 − (5.68 × age)
Women: RMR = 447 + (3.1 × ht. in cm) + (9.2 × wt. in kg)
 − (4.33 × age)

Example: Bob is a thirty-two-year-old male who is 6 feet tall and weighs 160 pounds:

88.36 + (4.8 × 183) + (13.4 × 72kg) − (5.68 × 32) = 1750

Alternate: Nearly as reliable, consider 1 calorie/kilogram body weight/hour × 24 hours:

160-pound athlete
160/2.2 = 72 kg
72 kg × 1 × 24 = 1,745 calories for RMR

To then estimate total caloric expenditure, multiply your RMR by one of the activity factors below.

RMR × 1.5 = weight maintenance for light exercisers
RMR × 1.8 = weight maintenance for moderately active people
 (up to 1 hour per day of activity)
RMR × 2.0 = weight maintenance for athletes exercising over an
 hour per day
RMR × 2.4 = weight maintenance for endurance athletes
 ——————— Total Daily Energy Expenditure

Finally, subtract calories to determine your desired rate of weight loss.

subtract 500 calories = ——————— for about a pound per week
 weight loss
subtract 1,000 calories = ——————— to lose about two pounds per
 week

Step Two: Determine Protein Requirements

When actively losing weight, it's best to obtain double the protein requirement of the RDA of .8 gram per kilogram (.36 gram per pound). When losing weight, strive to have 1.6 to 1.8 grams per kilogram or .7 to .8 gram of protein per pound. Also, it has been found that higher-quality proteins rich in essential amino acids may offer additional benefits to incomplete protein sources.

Step Three: Determine Carbohydrate Requirements

As an athlete, carbohydrates are required to sustain physical activity and your central nervous system. During times of weight loss, it's okay to reduce carbohydrates to 5 to 6 grams per kilogram from 8 to 10 grams per kilogram or during times of intense training.

Step Four: Determine Fat Requirements

Once you calculate how much protein and carbohydrates are needed, the remainder of your daily calories should come from fat. In many cases, fat will be less than 20 percent of calories.

Step Five: Use the Eating-for-Energy Meal Suggestions in Chapter 11

This will help ensure that you are getting the appropriate calories.

Step Six: Include High-Quality Protein (Eggs, Meat, Poultry, Seafood) at Meals Whenever Possible

Research suggests that the essential amino acids and branched chain amino acids are best for muscle-sparing, protein-stimulating benefits. In addition, protein is satiating, so it helps to keep you fuller longer to help curb your appetite.

Step Seven: After Training, within an Hour Try to Get In Some Type of Protein Rich in Essential Amino Acids

One study found that providing 6 grams of essential amino acids in a beverage after resistance training helped athletes retain muscle mass. Nine amino acids are generally regarded as essential for humans: isoleucine, leucine, lysine, threonine, tryptophan, methionine, histidine, valine, and phenylalanine.

Step Eight: Don't Skip Meals

Some studies have found that when athletes lose weight, the more they can keep energy intake matched to expenditure, the easier it is to lose body fat. For example, those who had the biggest variation in calorie intake (huge meals, then skipping meals) were more likely to have a higher percentage of body fats.

Step Nine: Eat a Healthy, Fiber-Rich Breakfast

Breakfast eaters have lower BMIs than do morning meal skippers. Research shows that breakfasts that are fiber rich (e.g., oats) may help with fat losses over sugary breakfasts.

Step Ten: Keep Weight Loss to No More Than a Pound or Two per Week Whenever Possible

As the rate of weight loss increases, so too does the percentage of fat-free mass (water, muscle, glycogen) that's lost, regardless of how much protein you consume.

Step Eleven: Continue to Train

Both aerobic and strength training offer benefits for optimizing body composition during times of caloric restriction.

Step Twelve: Consume Adequate Amounts of Carbohydrates before, during, and after Your Training

This will help compensate for the low muscle glycogen stores that will result from being in energy deficit as you lose weight.

Metabolic Rate: Fact versus Fiction

Our metabolic rate is like the engine of an automobile, but our engines must work 24/7 to keep us alive. Some people have a Hemi under the hood, while others are more like Hybrids. Athletes have a keen interest in their metabolic rate or resting energy expenditure because it can help them determine their energy needs to lose, maintain, or even gain weight.

What Is Metabolic Rate?

Your metabolic rate is measured as either the basal metabolic rate (BMR) or resting metabolic rate (RMR). The BMR is usually measured in the morning after an overnight fast and lying down for thirty minutes, whereas the RMR is often measured in the afternoon, several hours after eating. It generally provides a result that is 10 to 20 percent higher than the BMR. Both values are often used interchangeably to describe how much energy your body needs to sustain itself.

The RMR or BMR represents about two-thirds of your total daily energy needs. Muscle movement (exercise, fidgeting, walking, daily activities) represents about 23 percent of total energy expenditure in the average American, while the thermic effect of food (effects of turning food into usable energy and waste in the body) represents another 10 percent. Very active individuals can match their RMR or surpass it with calories expended from energy.

Do Thinner People Have Higher Metabolic Rates?

Nope. The opposite is true. One effective way to increase your metabolic rate is to gain weight. That's because both fat and muscle require energy to sustain themselves. And for every pound you gain, one-quarter of it is generally lean tissue. The opposite is true when you lose weight: each pound lost includes 25 percent or more lean tissue.

Research shows that for every pound lost, your body requires about ten fewer calories. Lose ten pounds and you now need to cut a hundred calories from your diet or exercise an additional hundred calories or you'll gain weight. This is part of the reason why weight maintenance is so much more challenging than losing weight.

Doesn't Exercise (Aerobic or Strength Training) Raise the Metabolic Rate Post-Exercise?

While this was once thought to be true, more recent research suggests that endurance athletes, such as marathoners and triathletes, have a few hours or even days after their events where their RMR is elevated; but for most athletes, the increase in RMR post-exercise is not enough to get excited about.

Even highly trained athletes often have RMR equal to their sedentary counterparts. While exercise is great for total energy expenditure, and is good for your heart and cardiovascular system and has many other health benefits, increasing metabolic rate is not one of the major benefits of exercise.

Does Adding Muscle Mass Increase Metabolic Rate?

Compared to fat tissue, muscle mass is more metabolically active. But in comparison to organs, your muscles are like a Hybrid while your organs are gas-guzzling V8s. Muscles burn about 13 kilocalories per kilogram per day, fat burns 4.5 kilocalories per kilogram per day, but organs burn 200 to 400 kilocalories per kilogram per day. In the end, your organs represent 60 to 70 percent of your metabolic rate, and muscles represent 16 to 22 percent.

And the most pounds of muscle mass that most unaided athletes can add in a year, 4 to 5 pounds of muscle, would add a need for 28 to 50 kilocalories per day or 7 to 10 kilocalories for each pound of muscle you gain.

Should I Have My BMR or RMR Measured?

If you are trying to lose weight, it's probably not a bad idea to get your RMR measured. Most health clubs now offer on-site metabolic rate tests.

At the very least, it will probably tell you that your weight woes are not due to low metabolism. Use the calculations we provided in this chapter for a fairly accurate measure of your RMR.

Top Ten Tips to Win at Losing from Top Athletes

1. Don't try any fad, crash, or omission-style diets. Stick with a balanced approach of more unprocessed, high-fiber foods: plenty of complex carbohydrates, lean protein, and healthy fats. For a plan, use the Energy to Burn guidelines in chapter 11.
2. Find your motivator (a photo of your too-large self, tight pants, schedule a nude photo shoot of yourself, reward yourself with a new piece of equipment when you reach your goal).
3. Use the preseason as your calorie-zapping time to lose weight.
4. Eat smaller, more frequent meals instead of two or three larger meals.
5. Organize your kitchen so that healthy foods are visible, and make it difficult to get to the more indulgent items. Or better yet, don't bring binge foods home.
6. Diet at night. It's easier to sleep through hunger than to be awake through it.
7. To get the scale to budge, keep a food log by writing down everything you eat or drink for three or four days.
8. Fuel yourself adequately before and during exercise so you don't have postexercise pig-outs.
9. Limit liquid calories. Drink more water and other calorie-free beverages, and save the sports drinks for when you're training or racing.
10. Get on the scale. Better yet, have your spouse, partner, or friend weigh you weekly (just like a 4-H piglet).

Fifty Ways to Lose up to Ten Pounds without Dieting

Since a pound of fat equals thirty-five hundred calories, if you try one of these tips every day this year you'll be roughly ten pounds lighter this time next year. That can take you from chub to champ, schlub to stud.

1. Eat three bites less. Have just three bites less during your meals or when eating out, and you'll save yourself a hundred calories.

2. Eat your calories, don't drink 'em. Because the body doesn't compensate for calories from liquids as well as it does from foods you chew, make a mental note of how many calorie-laden drinks you're downing. Replace just eight ounces of soda a day with water or a calorie-free beverage and you'll be ten pounds lighter in a year.

3. Keep TV watching to less than two hours per day.

4. Invest in nonstick sprays and pans for cooking. You'll save a hundred calories for every tablespoon of oil or butter you don't use.

5. Turn your back to the buffet table at parties so you can't be tempted by what you see; you'll save yourself a hundred or more calories.

6. Cut sugar by a third in all recipes; use applesauce or prune puree to replace half the fat in baked goods. You can replace 100 percent of the fat with applesauce in brownies or a moist cake and they'll still come out great.

7. Substituting fruit or veggies for a piece of candy once daily will save you more than a hundred calories. Also, the fiber in the produce will help keep you to feel full longer.

8. Drink from tall, thin glasses. Research from the University of Illinois found that consumers drink, on average, 77 percent more when they drink out of short, squat glasses compared to tall, thin glasses. The amount of liquid calories is perceived as less when served in a short, wide glass.

9. Why sit when you can stand? Don't despair when you can't get a seat on the C train or you're stuck in the DMV line. Standing for fifty minutes daily equals a hundred calories.

10. Downsize your plates and bowls. Seriously. If you eat out of large containers or from large plates, you're going to eat more calories—probably much more than a hundred calories.

11. Watch your "healthy" meals. Research shows that when consumers ate at Subway, they ate 31 percent more calories compared to when they go to a fast-food restaurant such as McDonald's. Cornell researchers said that eating at healthier restaurants often prompts us to order high-calorie sides, such as chips and soda.

12. Eat breakfast. No matter what it is, people who eat breakfast consume fewer calories in total during the day. Ideally, you want to have three meals and two snacks daily. That helps keep your energy levels up and keeps you from getting ravenous from not eating for long periods of time.

13. Sleep more. There's a reason it's called "beauty" sleep. Research shows that extra sleep can help people stick with healthier eating and helps control hormones that trigger food cravings.

14. Move during TV commercials. If you walk around, march in place, or do simple calisthenics during TV commercials, you'll burn at least a hundred calories during your two-hour TV limit.

15. Instead of drinking a twenty-ounce bottle of soda, fruit juice, or other sweetened beverage at one time, make it last for two and a half servings (as the label states). Dilute it with water or seltzer if you need to drink more.

16. Add a half-hour, low-intensity workout first thing in the morning before you eat breakfast.

17. Add one cross-training session to your routine each week.

18. Clean the house, shovel snow, or rake the leaves for just thirty minutes.

19. Choose plain, nonfat yogurt or artificially sweetened containers of it over fruit-flavored and you can save up to a hundred calories per eight-ounce serving.

20. Eat your fruit fresh, not dried. Snack on ten grapes instead of a mini-box of raisins and you'll save yourself a hundred calories.

21. Walk your dog (or take your neighbor's). You'll burn about 6.5 calories per minute of walking your dog. That's 100 calories for a 15-minute walk.

22. Add a salad before lunch. New research shows that a large salad before a meal saves 125 calories for that meal. Add a salad to every lunch and lose 12 pounds in a year!

23. Eat, then go food shopping. Think of today's supermarkets and specialty markets as goodie factories with samples galore. Eat before shopping so you can avoid the temptation of tasting the samples. It also will help you from bringing home indulgent items.

24. Don't drown your salad in dressing. Swap your regular bottled dressing for fat-free and save more than a hundred calories per two-tablespoon serving.

25. Nosh lightly. Munch on two ounces of baked potato or tortilla chips instead of their traditional full-fat counterparts. Each two-ounce nosh will save you a hundred calories.

26. Skip the dip or lighten it up. Instead of having guacamole with your

favorite chips, try salsa. You'll save more than a hundred calories per quarter cup.

27. Order a virgin (mixed drink, that is). A virgin cocktail will save you about a hundred calories, since the distilled spirits pack in a hundred calories per ounce-and-a-half shot of distilled spirits.

28. Substitute two cans of low-carb or light beer for regular and you'll save a hundred calories.

29. Skip the cheese on your sandwich or next burger. An ounce of cheese packs in a hundred calories.

30. Have a whole-wheat English muffin or two slices of whole-wheat toast instead of a bagel for breakfast. You'll save more than 150 calories.

31. Simplify cocktails. Having wine, champagne, beer, or spirits with noncalorie beverages can save more than a hundred calories per drink. Fancy mixed drinks such as Margaritas, Brandy Alexanders, and Sea Breezes can pack in three hundred calories or more per drink.

32. Eat three a day—of nonfat or low-fat dairy foods, that is. Research shows that individuals who eat more dairy foods are leaner than their dairy-eschewing counterparts. Scientists believe that components in dairy products help speed fat metabolism while helping the body build muscle mass.

33. Choose the best licks. Skip super-premium ice cream and have a frozen fruit juice bar to save a hundred calories.

34. Get off the subway one or two stops earlier, suggests personal trainer Eddie Carrington of Bally Total Fitness. The fifteen- to twenty-block walk will equal about a hundred calories, and you'll get a chance to enjoy the scenery and do some window shopping while you burn calories.

35. Carrington also suggests getting a move on at work. Instead of e-mailing, walk to coworkers for their input. And walk to get your lunch instead of having it delivered.

36. Replenish your glass of regular soda with diet soda, water, or seltzer and you'll save a hundred calories for eight ounces.

37. Nuts are nutritious but high in calories. Eat about fifteen fewer mixed nuts than normal to shave off a hundred calories.

38. Eat the bread, not the butter. Just one tablespoon of butter with the breadbasket equals a hundred calories.

39. For a hearty breakfast, enjoy a hearty bowl of whole-grain oats, one of the most satiating breakfast options.

40. Limit your bedtime snack to a bowl of cereal with skim milk to avoid excess calories from snack foods.

41. Order half a deli sandwich instead of a whole one. Most deli sandwiches pack in more than five hundred calories. Eat half the sandwich and a piece of fruit instead of the other half and save yourself two hundred calories.

42. Enjoy a lettuce pita pocket sandwich. Have a sandwich wrapped in large red leaf lettuce instead of pita to save more than 150 calories.

43. Eat three squares and two to three snacks per day. People who eat more frequently while dieting experience a less pronounced reduction in metabolic rate.

44. Swap a heaping plate of steamed vegetables for the same amount of starchy carbs such as pasta or rice.

45. Change your coffee break. Ask for skim versus whole milk for your grande (sixteen ounces), skip the whipped cream on your Starbucks drinks, or downsize from a venti to a grande or a grande to a tall. Some coffee drinks can pack in more calories than two glazed doughnuts.

46. At fast-food restaurants, order the smallest hamburger without cheese instead of the larger, specialty burgers. A McDonald's hamburger instead of a Quarter Pounder will shave 150 calories off your meal.

47. Downsize the fries. Order one size smaller than you normally do to attack your own fat.

48. Chocoholic? Have a bag of Raisinets instead of a gooey candy bar to satisfy your chocolate craving while saving a hundred calories.

49. At work or home, keep goodies such as chocolates or hard candy in a drawer or several feet away and out of sight. University of Illinois researchers found that if you keep candy in reach at work, you'll eat, on average, two more pieces (fifty to a hundred calories) than if the candy is farther away. Think out of sight, out of mouth.

50. If you're using a sports bar as a between-meal nosh, eat half instead of all of it.

3

Carbohydrates:
The Ultimate Fuel Source

Five items always in your cupboard: "raisins, oatmeal, canned tomatoes, rice, canned organic vegetable soups."
—*Barry Burr, PowerBar Team elite athlete*

Cut Out Carb Confusion

Like low-waist denim jeans or men with long hair, carbohydrates fall in and out of favor. The carb-cutting craze hit big in the late 1990s, but if you track the history, this trend had recurred over the years, popping up in new diet books, with novel names, every other decade. It is likely that the trend will return, but after reading this chapter, you should be unscathed when it presents on bookshelves, diet blogs, and quack sites. The aim is that you leave with a clear understanding of what carbohydrate-containing foods are, what constitutes a carbohydrate, why you need them, how many grams you should include, and most importantly, how they influence your performance as an active person. We want to put the carb confusion to rest and leave you with the clarity you need to enjoy a whole-grain baguette, side of brown rice, or veggie-topped pasta dish.

Due to the popularity of the Atkins Diet and the low-carbohydrate revolution of the 1970s, carbohydrates have

"I totally lost weight on the low-carb diet! I was diligent and disciplined. I cut out all carbs from fruits to alcohol. My total weight loss was twenty-six pounds and I was very pleased . . . until I woke up with more hair on my pillow than my head. My doctor said one thing to me when he ordered my blood work: 'Eat carbs again.'"

—*anonymous dieter testimonial*

earned a reputation as indulgent, "fattening," and even unnecessary to your diet. The low-carb craze was rekindled again during the 1990s with the popularity of similar diets, such as the South Beach Diet. We recognize the appeal of these diets in an age of widespread overweight and obesity. Low-carbohydrate diets purport to offer a simple solution to a complex problem—managing our weight in an environment where cheap, high-calorie food is widely available. Such diets try to simplify what can only truly be achieved through the hard work of incorporating a balanced diet and regular exercise into our lifestyle.

It is worth addressing low-carbohydrate diet claims in this book because many people, including athletes, follow such diets for some period of time to improve their appearance or to "make" a certain weight for their sport. For some people, especially those who dieted unsuccessfully in the past, the promises of such diets are more convincing than the scientific evidence showing the limitations and potential dangers of these diets.

You Will Lose Weight

To acknowledge what you may have heard or experienced, some people will lose a few pounds during the first few days on a low-carbohydrate diet. These first few pounds are a combination of water weight lost when carbohydrates are restricted, and a small amount of fat loss from eating fewer overall calories. After all, the strictest of the low-carbohydrate diets essentially bans foods from four of the six major food groups; thus there is not much left to choose from.

However, within a short time the dieter often notices the number on the scale climbing back upward. This is because, for one, when you start adding carbs back into the diet, water returns to the cells. Because water is heavy in the body, its reentry is reflected as weight gain. Next, food restriction slows metabolism; thus, when calorie intake returns to normal, body mass is regained quickly. And finally, after a period of restriction, an increased urge to indulge in carbohydrate foods also may lead to a rapid weight rebound.

These are the scientific reasons why low-carbohydrate diets do not work in the long run. There have been a number of studies on the effects of low-carbohydrate diets. A recent comprehensive literature review published in *Current Opinion in Gastroenterology* summarized the current research, stating that the long-term weight loss of low-carbohydrate dieters is not significantly different from that of dieters who follow low-fat diets.

The authors advise caution against low-carbohydrate diets based on a lack of data on the long-term health effects, especially their effects on the heart and blood vessels. Furthermore, there have been few studies on the effects of carbohydrates beyond the six-month point, yet we know that complications of cardiovascular disease and other adverse health conditions often take a number of years to reach detectable levels in the average person.

But Carbs Make You Fat . . . Right?

Moreover, the major premise behind low-carbohydrate diets—that carbohydrates promote weight gain more than other nutrients—is false. There is nothing magical about protein or fat, just as there is nothing evil about carbohydrates. None of these nutrients causes weight gain or weight loss on its own, since overall calorie consumption versus calories burned determines weight. Eating more calories than your body will burn, calories from any food or combination of foods, can cause weight gain. Approximately thirty-five hundred calories, whether they are consumed as popcorn, steak, butter, or broccoli, will cause an individual to gain one pound of weight.

- Carbohydrates provide four calories per gram.
- Protein provides four calories per gram.
- Fat provides nine calories per gram.

A recent meta-analysis, a report that synthesizes and summarizes data from a number of good studies in the literature, supports the notion that calories, not carbohydrates, count in terms of body weight. The study examined the effects of low-carbohydrate diets, finding that weight loss was linked to three factors: decreased caloric intake, increased length of diet period, and higher initial body weight of study subjects.

Low-Carb—Crazy if You're Active

There also has been research on low-carbohydrate diets and athletic performance. Rosenkranz et al. reported on low-carbohydrate diets in the *International Journal of Sports Nutrition, Exercise, and Metabolism* in June 2007. A group of athletes was divided and assigned to follow one of two diets: a low-carbohydrate diet or the recommended grain-based diet. The athletes on the low-carbohydrate diet experienced disruptions in their training schedule, higher heart rates, and higher perceived rates of exertion during exercise. Blood tests showed the low-carb dieters to have elevated total cholesterol and LDL levels.

Athletes should take heed of some potentially dangerous effects on the body that low-carbohydrate diets can pose. Some reported side effects include ketosis (elevated levels of ketone bodies—a type of fuel that comes from the breakdown of fat for fuel), fatigue, weakness, headaches, constipation, dizziness, and dehydration. None of these will improve performance. To make matters worse, a prolonged state of ketosis can damage the kidneys and disrupt the body's acid-base balance. Ketosis has been linked to electrolyte imbalances and disruption of heart rhythm.

Fat Adaptation?

So what about the effects of the high-fat intake associated with a diet such as the Atkins? A recent study looked at the effects of "fat adaptation," which is essentially a type of fat loading similar to the high-fat intakes of Atkins-like diets. Some athletes try fat adaptation to reduce glycogen use and increase fat burn during exercise, with the goal of enhancing and extending their speed and endurance. The results, reported in *International Sports Medicine*, suggest that even when athletes "fat-adapt" for five or six days before an event, their performance is not enhanced during endurance activities. The only group that may benefit, the authors speculate, may be ultra-endurance athletes who engage in events lasting more than four hours. They state that the differences among even elite athletes in terms of benefits makes formulating any general conclusions or recommendations very difficult.

The Truth

Nothing is gained by restricting quality carbohydrates. Carbohydrates are in some of the most nutritious foods on earth. Think about recently anointed "superfoods" such as bananas, beans, berries, broccoli, and green, leafy vegetables. Take bananas, for example. Dr. Atkins would summarily denounce this nutritious whole food as wholly fattening; South Beach may allow them, but only in carefully measured amounts. But bananas contain not only sugar, which is a carbohydrate, but also starches and fiber, nutrients that form the foundation of a healthful diet. Given what we know about saturated fat, trans fat, and heart disease, wouldn't we be better off limiting high-fat meats than limiting bananas?

Furthermore, cutting carbohydrates also means cutting many of the micronutrients in carbohydrate-rich foods, including a host of vitamins and minerals such as vitamins A and C, which repair oxidative damage to the tissues caused by exercise; the B vitamins, which are responsible for supporting energy production; and calcium, magnesium, potassium, iron, zinc, and other minerals that keep bones, blood, heart, and skeletal muscles healthy. You must ask yourself: without the micronutrients necessary to utilize food for energy, what good is any food?

Final Buzz Kill

A final point to consider about low-carbohydrate diets is that they are based on the assumption that the diet can be summarily and simplistically divided into good foods (protein and fat) and bad foods (carbohydrates). Such rigid, arbitrary rules detract from the pleasure and enjoyment that healthful eating should bring. The reality is that there is nothing simplistic about the diet, or any of the nutrients in it. Most foods are composed of many different types of nutrients, and any diet that suggests avoiding or severely limiting any of them should be avoided. No food should be avoided absolutely, and no food should be eaten in excess. Let the dietary guidelines, a tried-and-true if somewhat imperfect source, guide your food choices from each food group and help you to eat a well-balanced diet. And for goodness sake, enjoy your food!

What's a Carbohydrate?

We can name some carbs—bread, cereal, pasta, rice—but speaking scientifically, what is a carbohydrate? A carbohydrate, as defined by a food chemist, is an organic compound that contains carbon, hydrogen, and oxygen in a variety of combinations. Carbohydrates, which are primarily in plant foods and in trace amounts in animal foods, are sugar molecules with a one-to-one ratio of carbon to water. In fact, the name "carbohydrate" shows that each carbon molecule is "hydrated."

Carbohydrates can be as simple as a single molecule or as complex as a chain of hundreds of thousands of sugar molecules. To give a basic overview, carbohydrates can be divided into two types: simple (sugars) and complex (starches and fibers).

Simple Carbohydrates

Simple carbohydrates include monosaccharides (one-sugar molecules) and disaccharides (two-sugar molecules). Monosaccharides include glucose (commonly known as blood sugar), fructose (fruit sugar), and galactose (a kind of milk sugar). Disaccharides—which are always composed of glucose plus another monosaccharide—include maltose, sucrose (table sugar), and lactose (milk sugar).

SIMPLE CARBOHYDRATES		
Monosaccharides		**Disaccharides**
Glucose + Glucose	=	Maltose
Glucose + Fructose	=	Sucrose
Glucose + Galactose	=	Lactose

Simply Sugar

When you think of simple carbohydrates, often you'll think of candy or junk food, and actually, many "simple" carbs are wasted calories (except for fruit, of course). If there is a type of carbohydrate to limit, it's the added sugar in candy, soft drinks, and sweet snack foods. These offer calories—the same four calories per gram offered by any other type of carbohydrate—but little else in terms of nutrition. That's why we often call them "empty" calories.

Simple carbohydrates are rapidly digested, sometimes even in the mouth or soon after entering the stomach, and they may raise blood sugar rapidly. They tend to generate a quick rush (think "sugar rush") of energy, which usually is short-lived. Once the body uses the available glucose in the blood, blood sugar levels drop again, and you may be left feeling tired and depleted. This reaction may be due to the large insulin release that causes cells to take up and use glucose quickly. As an athlete, however, simple sugars aren't evil and are actually the fuel that sustains most endurance athletes as well as those in high-intensity sports. Since exercise suppresses insulin release, blood sugar levels remain fairly stable during exercise.

Better Sugar?

The sugar in honey or real maple syrup may contain a few more nutrients than regular table sugar, but the body processes the sugar in these foods in essentially the same way as it would the sugar in a candy bar. Therefore, even these foods and supposedly "healthy" sugars in real-fruit jams and jellies should be eaten in moderate amounts. Health authorities encourage the general couch-potato population to limit simple sugars (those listed as "sugars" on food labels) to 10 percent of daily calories, but athletes generally need more than 10 percent of their calories from sugars to fuel activity.

Sweet Substitutes

Sugar alternatives are often recommended for effective weight management, diabetes management, or simply as "healthier" alternatives to sugar. Artificial sweeteners such as saccharine, aspartame, and sucralose may help prevent dental caries by stimulating saliva production without causing the harmful plaque that sugar generates. Whether certain artificial sweeteners lead to health problems, or perhaps lead to overeating, are questions under study.

Aspartame

Aspartame is the most studied of the sweeteners, and it appears not to present a health threat. However, individuals with phenylketonuria (PKU) can become ill from digesting aspartame because it contains the amino acid phenylalanine. The makers of aspartame claim that it contributes four calories per gram, the same as table sugar.

Saccharine

Saccharine has been used for more than a century in the United States, but it has undergone scrutiny for potential cancer-causing effects. Today saccharine is still used in some tabletop sweeteners and beverages as well as in cosmetics and pharmaceutical products. Saccharine-containing products contain a special health warning. It contains zero calories.

Sucralose

Sucralose was approved by the FDA in 1998 and is the newest of the major artificial sweeteners. It is the only such product made from natural sugar, although the body does not recognize its molecular structure and passes it undigested through the digestive tract. It therefore has no calories.

Acesulfame-K

Acesulfame-K, approved in 1988, is another apparently safe sweetener used by itself to sweeten foods and beverages. It appears in a number of foods such as puddings, gelatins, baked goods, and alcoholic beverages.

Sweet Replacement

In addition, a number of artificial "sugar replacers" have entered the market. These reduced-calorie products, which appear in chewing gum and other products, are essentially sugar alcohols. They have names such as mannitol, sorbitol, zylitol, maltitol, isomalt, and lacitol. They are "sugar-free" but not "calorie-free." They contain two to three calories per gram.

It's a Complex Issue

Complex carbohydrates are formed by tens or even hundreds of glucose molecules linked together. Two of the most important complex carbohydrates for athletes to recognize are starches and fibers.

Starches are found most plentifully in grains such as rice, wheat, and oats, but also in tubers such as potatoes and in legumes such as beans. Starch is essentially the energy that plants store as their own energy source. When we eat starches, this plant energy becomes human energy. Our bodies break down plant starch to units of glucose that are sent to our blood and taken up by our cells, or stored in our liver or muscles in long chains called glycogen.

Net Carbs = No Meaning

"Net carbs" is a term coined by low-carbohydrate-diet-product manufacturers, not nutritionists. "Net carbs," often listed on the labels of foods marketed as low carbohydrate, usually refers to the total carbohydrates minus the carbohydrates from fiber and artificial sweeteners. These carbohydrates are assumed to be non-contributors to the overall calorie content since the body does not break them down in the same way and does not derive as many calories from them as it does from sugar. Whereas insoluble fiber has important health benefits, artificial sweeteners offer the body no known nutritional benefits. There is no approved definition or nutritious use for "net carbs."

Fill Up on Fiber

Fiber, another type of polysaccharide, acts as the skeleton of plants, giving them their structural integrity. Fibers are in virtually all fruits and vegetables and also in grains and legumes. There are even different types of fiber whose names probably will sound familiar.

Soluble Fiber

First, there is soluble fiber, which includes the gooey constituents of plants such as pectins and some hemicelluloses and mucilages. Soluble fiber is called such because it is soluble in water; it actually turns into a sort of gel, rather than remaining stringy and tough when mixed with water. Soluble fiber has been in health reports over the past several years for its digestion-slowing, cholesterol-lowering, and blood glucose-stabilizing effects. When you think of soluble fiber, think of fruits, oats, barley, and legumes.

Insoluble Fiber

Insoluble fiber, which you may know as "roughage," includes the tougher cellulose, hemicellulose, and lignans in plant foods such as bran (e.g., corn and wheat bran), whole grains, and vegetables (especially cabbage, carrots, and brussels sprouts). When you think about insoluble fiber, think about strings of celery or wheat bran. Insoluble fiber adds bulk to stool and therefore helps move waste quickly through the digestive tract. Scientists believe that it may help prevent gastrointestinal disorders by reducing strain and stress on the colon and rectum. Insoluble fiber also helps to slow starch hydrolysis and also may help delay glucose absorption in the same way soluble fiber can.

Insoluble fiber has other characteristics worth noting. First, it contains fewer calories than normal carbohydrates (about two calories per gram versus four calories per gram), since the body cannot break it down for energy as completely or as readily as it can other types of carbohydrates. Second, even trace amounts of insoluble fiber offer health benefits. When this type of fiber is broken down in the colon, it results in fatty acids that nourish colon cells and colonic bacteria, keeping the digestive tract healthy.

		Fiber Content		
Food Item	**Serving Size**	**Total Fiber (g)**	**Insoluble (g)**	**Soluble (g)**
Apples	1 small	3.9	1.6	2.3
Broccoli	½ cup cooked	2.7	1.4	1.3
Kidney beans	½ cup cooked	4.5	4.0	0.5
Lettuce	1 cup	0.5	0.3	0.2
Oatmeal	½ cup cooked	1.6	1.1	0.5
Oranges	1 medium	2.0	0.7	1.3
Popcorn	3 cups popped	2.8	2.0	0.8
Strawberries	¾ cup	2.4	1.5	0.9
Whole-wheat bread	1 slice	2.9	2.8	0.1
Zucchini	½ cup cooked	2.5	1.4	1.1

HIGH-FIBER FOODS

Give Your Menu a Fiber Makeover

It's pretty easy to give your menu a fiber makeover. You don't need to turn your kitchen upside down, nor do you need to lose the things you love. Here is an example of an easy, yummy menu makeover that will give you more fiber with all the good taste and convenience you need!

Low-Fiber Menu	High-Fiber Menu
Breakfast	*Breakfast*
1 cup Honey Bunches of Oats cereal	1 cup Honey Nut Cheerios cereal
½ cup skim milk	½ cup skim milk
1 cup orange juice	1 medium orange
Water	Water
Snack	*Snack*
1 cup pretzels	3 cups air-popped popcorn
Lunch	*Lunch*
Sandwich	Sandwich
2 slices white bread	2 slices whole-grain bread
3 ounces turkey breast	3 ounces turkey breast
1 ounce American cheese	1 ounce American cheese
1 small bag potato chips	1 cup baby carrots
1 medium banana	1 medium banana
1 cup skim milk	1 cup skim milk
Snack	*Snack*
Quaker Chocolate Chip Granola Bar	Fiber One chocolate chip cereal bar
Dinner	*Dinner*
4 ounces pork tenderloin	4 ounces pork tenderloin
1 small baked potato, skin not eaten	1 small baked potato, skin eaten
1 teaspoon soft spread	1 teaspoon soft spread
½ cup white rice	½ cup brown and wild rice mixture
½ cup green beans	½ cup green beans
Iced tea	Iced tea
Snack	*Snack*
2 tablespoons peanut butter	2 tablespoons peanut butter
8 crackers	8 pieces of celery
Nutrient Analysis	*Nutrient Analysis*
2,084 calories	1,726 calories
290 grams carbohydrates	232 grams carbohydrates
96 grams proteins	96 grams proteins
60 grams fats	46 grams fats
20 grams saturated fats	13 grams saturated fats
18 grams fiber	32 grams fiber

Feed Your Brain!

As the principal energy source for the body and the brain, carbohydrates are a critical component of the diet. Consuming ample carbohydrates is crucial for good general health and vital for top athletic performance. Let's go through carb sources and the recommendations for adding them to your diet.

Go Grain!

The 2005 Dietary Guidelines for Americans and MyPyramid.gov make complex carbohydrates the foundation of your diet.

MyPyramid encourages us to choose six to ten servings of grains per day, with the higher end of this range for active people.

A serving, which is defined differently for specific foods, is different from a portion. Most people eat portions of foods such as bread, rice, or pasta that far exceed the amount that the creators of the national guidelines had in mind. For example, a serving of grain equals one slice of bread, a quarter bagel, half a cup of cooked rice or pasta, or half a cup of ready-to-eat cereal. By contrast, consider the average restaurant-size "portion" of pasta; it often equals five or more "servings."

Focus on Whole Grains

The Dietary Guidelines also recommend that we make at least half of the grain servings we consume whole grains. Examples of whole grains include brown rice, whole-grain pasta, and steel-cut oats. The difference between whole grains and processed grains is that whole grains have not undergone milling or processing to strip away their outer layer. They thereby retain the bran, fiber, and any vitamins and minerals naturally packaged within that layer. When you seek out whole-grain foods, look for a label indicating "100% whole wheat." Manufacturers are permitted to make claims such as "contains whole grains," but this does not ensure that most of the grains in the product are whole. Pick from the following to add some whole grain to your day:

- Baked goods made with whole-grain flour
  - Whole-grain bread
  - Whole-grain rolls
  - Whole-grain sandwich buns
  - Whole-grain tortillas

- Brown rice
- Buckwheat
- Bulgur (cracked wheat)
- Cereal
- Cheerios
- Raisin Bran
- Oatmeal
- Popcorn
- Whole-grain pasta
- Wild rice

Also on the grocery shelf, white bread and most sweetened breakfast cereals contain largely processed grains that have been bleached and treated with colorings and preservatives. Much of the nutritional value is lost in food processing and then sometimes sprayed on afterward. Thus, when you do choose processed grains, try to choose fortified ones. The main disadvantages of eating only processed grains is that you will miss out on fiber, and a number of naturally occurring vitamins and minerals, as well as the natural oils in the bran layer.

Eat Your Veggies

Vegetables also are nutritious, carbohydrate-rich foods that contain mainly starch and fiber. In addition, vegetables are packed with vitamins and minerals, such as the antioxidant vitamins A and C, as well as vitamins B and K and the minerals potassium and calcium. Vegetables also contain an abundance of phytochemicals such as lutein, for example, which has been shown to support healthy eyesight. Research on the various phytochemicals in fruits and vegetables is just beginning, and scientists believe that there is something about eating whole fruits and vegetables (instead of taking nutritional supplements) that give us major health benefits (visit the chapter on supplements and functional foods for more on that). We don't need to mention the thousands of studies that have shown that fruits and vegetables can help prevent chronic diseases such as type 2 diabetes, cardiovascular disease, and a variety of cancers—just remember what your mother said.

The current recommendation for vegetable intake is 2½ cups per day. This recommendation was formerly expressed in terms of servings, but in the most recent MyPyramid.gov, cups replaced servings to help consumers better visualize a proper serving. However, a "cup" is not always a cup as you know it. For example, two cups of leafy greens equals a one-cup serving of vegetables. This is because you need to eat more lettuce than, say, broccoli (for which one cup *is* actually a one-cup serving) to get equal amounts of nutrients and calories. As a rule, count on one cup of most vegetables equaling a one-cup serving, except for salad-type, leafy greens.

To get your 2½ cups of vegetables, you can eat 1 cup of broccoli, 1 cup of red peppers, and ½ cup of spinach. Or you can eat 5 servings of ½ cup of any veggies you wish.

Color Me Healthy

According to the dietary guidelines, it is also important to focus on variety in color. It's best to eat green, yellow, orange, and red vegetables, aiming for the most variety possible every day.

For those who say "I don't like vegetables," we would argue that there are so many different flavors and tastes in the veggie family, how could this be? We think a little creativity is in order. There are more types of vegetables in today's supermarkets, farm stands, and farmer's markets than ever before. Let's try a clever approach to veggies:

- Try some flavor enhancements, such as cutting vegetables and eating them raw with light dips such as yogurt and dill, or soy sauce and low-fat cream cheese.

- You also can give vegetables a whole new flavor by grilling or sautéing them with a small amount of olive oil, or seasoning with Mrs. Dash.

- You may want to try one of the many types of vegetable juices on the market or prepare your own in a blender, since several different flavors merged may make certain vegetables more appealing to you. (The same is true for fruit.)

- Try seasonal delights! Another way to get vegetables with appealing flavor is to eat the ones in season locally. If you live in the Northeast and it's winter, eat root vegetables such as sweet potatoes and turnips. If it's summer, go for cucumbers, peppers, and squash. Your year-round selection will probably be much wider if you live in a more temperate climate. But wherever you live, seek out new vegetables and ways to prepare them whenever possible to change your repertoire.

- Most people prefer the taste of fresh vegetables over frozen or canned. Try all types to see what you like. And remember, as we get older (even if you don't call yourself "old"), tastes change! Just because you didn't like asparagus as a kid doesn't necessarily mean you won't like it as an adult.

Beans Make You Healthy

Legumes are another excellent source of starch and fiber. Some legumes, such as black beans, have up to seven grams of fiber per serving. Eating legumes helps make significant headway toward meeting the current daily fiber recommendation of twenty to thirty-five grams. And beans and peas are loaded with nutrients, including iron and zinc. Many cultures have relied for centuries on the complete nutrition provided by beans and rice and have enjoyed low cardiovascular disease and cancer rates largely because of it.

Beans are very versatile; they can be eaten as a main or side dish, or sprinkled on salad, pureed and eaten as a sauce, or added to soups and stews. In terms of variety, today's bean choices are impressive. Take a peek; they are all healthful, flavorful, widely available, and easy to prepare:

- Black beans
- Kidney beans
- Chickpeas (garbanzo beans)
- White beans
- Green beans
- Baked beans
- Soybeans (affectionately called edamame)

Fruits

Fruits contain simple sugars as well as starch and fiber. Unlike "junk" foods that contain only simple sugars, fruits offer much more than sweetness. Vitamins A and C, potassium, and fiber are just a few of the valuable nutrients in large quantities in fruits. In fact, fruit is an excellent snack for athletes who need to increase their carbohydrate intake. Fruit offers a refreshing taste, a high water content that helps with hydration, and low-calorie, yet filling, nourishment. Fruits are often well tolerated and most are portable, with their edible portions protected by their own natural skins or peels. To get the freshest-tasting fruit, try to eat what's in season.

Many people, including many athletes, do not get the recommended amount of fruit servings per day. MyPyramid recommends two cups of fruit per day, which can be met by eating two whole fruits such as one small apple, one large banana or a large orange, or four half-cup servings of canned or dried fruit. One eight-ounce cup of 100 percent fruit juice also counts as a cup of fruit.

However, if you enjoy fruit juice, caution is in order. First, the label stating "100% fruit juice" is important. Drinks with labels that say "contains real juice" or "all natural" do not ensure that the juice actually comes from real fruit. Second, it is important to try not to take in too many calories from juice. Research shows that when calories are sipped and not eaten, individuals tend to feel less satisfied and tend to overconsume fluids and subsequently calories. This can be particularly true for sweetened drinks that contain little or no fiber.

Make Your Carbs Count

As you can glean from the information above, carbohydrates come in many varieties, from extremely nutritious to essentially nutritionally void. When it comes to calories versus nutrition, the carbohydrates to include in the diet are whole grains, vegetables, and fruits. Vegetables and fruits in particular are nutrient-dense "calorie bargains." This means that people can eat a large volume of these foods and derive a lot of good nutrition from them without a lot of calories.

Barbara Rolls of Penn State University coined the term "volumetrics" to describe a way of eating that focuses on satisfying hunger through low-calorie, high-nutrient foods. Because fruits and vegetables have high water and fiber contents, they tend to make us feel full quickly. Thus we end up feeling full after eating a large volume in terms of mass but not in terms of calories. Carbohydrates (and protein) contain four calories per gram, versus the nine calories per gram in fat. Thus we can eat a greater amount of fruits and vegetables than we can of fatty foods and still manage our weight.

On the other hand, there are carbohydrates that are best eaten in small amounts. The ones to limit are highly processed, sweet, or salty snack foods such as potato chips, crackers, and cookies. These foods may provide some energy in terms of calories, but these calories usually are from fat. In addition, they usually provide few vitamins or minerals. Since, calorie for calorie, these foods offer little nutrition, we consider them nutrient-poor, energy-dense foods. It is also easy to overeat such foods because they contain little fiber. And because they often contain lots of calories, overeating junk food can quickly lead to weight gain.

A volumetrics-type plan is good for most people, since most people like to know that they can eat a fair amount of food without "getting fat." It also can work for athletes as long as they get enough overall calories to satisfy their higher-than-average energy needs. Athletes concerned about managing their weight are better off following a philosophy such as volumetrics than a low-carbohydrate diet. A diet high in fruits and vegetables can help them stay hydrated and obtain the lasting energy they need to carry out the physical demands of sports training or competition.

Putting Carbs to Work

How does our whole-wheat bagel and side of strawberries turn into usable energy? In an effort to educate and hopefully not bore you, we'd like to give you a little carb digestion 101 so you understand how the food you eat fuels you.

Carb Digestion 101

When we eat carbohydrate-containing foods, they are broken down by various enzymes in the digestive tract. This process begins at the mouth and does not end completely until food enters the colon, at which time there is not much left except fiber. The simple sugars in foods are broken down by gastric and intestinal enzymes, and then enter the bloodstream as glucose. The more complex carbohydrate molecules are broken down into glucose molecules in the stomach and intestines. Glucose travels in the blood and, when insulin is released from the pancreas, the cells take it up for energy.

Storing Your Energy

Glucose has multiple destinies in the body. Not only is it used within the cells for energy, but if there is more sugar in the blood than the body can use at once, glucose can be converted to storage forms. One storage form is fat, stored in adipose cells. This is not the body's preferred pathway for glucose, however, because making glucose into fat is an energy-expensive process. The body would prefer to use glucose as it is or else store it in its other, more readily usable form—glycogen.

Glycogen is to humans as starch is to plants; it is our go-to energy source. Glycogen is formed of long chains of glucose, and it resides in the liver and in muscle tissue, where it can be used directly upon breakdown.

When we begin exercising, the body will use fat and glucose available in the bloodstream, and then tap fat stores for fuel. Next, as the energy demands of exercise increase, the body will begin breaking down glycogen molecules into individual glucose molecules and sending these to the blood to be used by muscles and other tissues.

When glycogen is depleted, the body continues to burn a certain amount of fat, but it also will continue to look for carbohydrates to sustain energy for physical activity. This is why it is important to be well fueled with carbohydrates before exercise or competition, and to snack lightly on carbohydrate-rich foods during all physical activity of considerable duration.

Although fat is the first fuel the body uses during a workout, carbohydrates are quickly drawn upon to provide energy at higher levels of speed and intensity.

As mentioned above, due to the water they contain, carbohydrates are heavy. This can be observed not only in the initial weight loss following a low-carbohydrate diet, but also when athletes "carb-load," or eat large portions of carbohydrate-rich foods to fuel for training or competition. (During this temporary, precompetition period, the athlete may eat enough carbohydrates to meet or exceed recommended carbohydrate intake.)

Most sources, including the American College of Sports Medicine, recommend that all healthy, nondiabetic individuals consume 55 to 65 percent of their daily calories from carbohydrates. For active people, it's about 2.3 to 3.2 grams per pound of body weight on light training days, 3.2 to 4.5 grams per pound for the heavy training days. (We will discuss this recommendation in food terms and personalize it for you later in this chapter.)

Carbs for the Female Athlete

Research reported in *Sports Medicine* and other scientific journals shows that female athletes are at greater risk of running a carbohydrate deficit than their male counterparts. A recent review of the literature shows that women are more likely to chronically or at least periodically restrict carbohydrates to achieve low body fat levels. This is particularly true for female endurance athletes and women competing in sports that place particular emphasis on a lean frame, such as figure skating or gymnastics.

A severe energy deficit in women can lead to the development of iron-deficiency anemia. It also can cause a drop in estrogen levels that disrupts the menstrual cycle and causes increased bone attrition. These conditions result because when the body enters a state of semi-starvation, it channels energy away from reproduction to provide fuel for vital functions. Scientists refer to this phenomenon of overexercising and undereating and the related health implications as the "female athlete triad." (This name seems to suggest that this kind of condition affects only women, although a similar form can affect men.) This condition can have dangerous, irreversible consequences, including infertility and osteoporosis. Usually, however, the condition can be ameliorated by increasing calorie intake to more completely meet energy demands.

Carb Ranking . . . Glycemic Index

For a number of years, particularly since the 1980s, when rates of overweight and obesity in the United States began to climb rapidly, experts have been concerned by the effects of different foods on appetite and blood sugar regulation. Scientists became interested in how different foods affect blood sugar, insulin release, and, in turn, energy usage and fat storage. In exploring the impact of foods on blood sugar, scientists constructed the glycemic index (GI), a scale for measuring and classifying foods based on how quickly they raise blood sugar. The best foods, according to these scientists, are foods that rank low on the index: foods that are digested slowly, cause a gradual rise in blood sugar, and lead to a moderate insulin response. The least favorable foods in terms of glucose response are those that elevate blood sugar levels quickly and lead to a rapid insulin response that results in a burst of energy that drops off rapidly.

Using the GI doesn't play much of a role in sports nutrition according to the research, despite the water-cooler chatter. Many experts have criticized the GI for a number of reasons, including reference foods not being well-defined and variations in foods that are often culture-dependent.

According to scientists, the cons for using the GI include:

- It is not applicable to exercising individuals, since the tests are conducted at rest and in a fasted state.
- GI tests actually show a high rate of variability of more than 30 percent, between individuals, and within the same individual.
- Studies have not consistently shown any performance benefit in consuming low- versus high-GI foods before, during, or after exercise.
- It is an unreliable and impractical way of measuring foods and making recommendations to athletes.

- The GI of a food varies from person to person and even in a single individual from day to day, depending on blood glucose levels, insulin resistance, and other factors.
- The GI is not the same as rate of digestion and absorption, which has a greater impact on athlete performance and GI distress during exercise.
- Once you mix foods together, the GI is invalidated, since foods are all mixed in the digestion process.

Research at the Australian Institute of Sport, in conjunction with researchers at Deakin University and the University of Melbourne, has examined the use of the GI in sports. Here's a summary of their findings:

- The jury is still out on the use of the GI in sports. It should not be used, and is not intended to be the overall ranking system, for carbohydrates. Foods should be selected to meet a variety of criteria based on taste, tolerance, convenience, and nutritional value.
- There is not enough evidence to recommend use of low GI foods prior to prolonged exercise. The best practice is to enlist your fueling strategies during exercise to avoid depleting your muscles' fuel supplies. You are better off using foods that are tried and true. Both high- and low-glycemic foods can work just fine.
- A very small percentage of the population (about 5 percent) have a condition called rebound hypoglycemia. For those individuals, a lower GI meal before exercise may be a better option.
- For prolonged exercise, athletes should consume carbohydrate during the event to fuel active muscles and thereby enhance performance. The choice of carbohydrate type seems to be more related to gut tolerance, hydration requirements, type of sport, previous experience, and individual tastes.
- There is some evidence that moderate and high-glycemic foods appear to help glycogen recovery after exercise compared to low-glycemic foods. The reason is not clearly understood. It is more important for the athlete to have adequate total carbohydrate intake than a specific glycemic index of food, with practicality being emphasized.

Research on the GI is preliminary at present for use with weight control. There is some evidence that limiting high-GI foods can be helpful for weight control in some people, perhaps those with a predisposition for overweight or obesity. The GI also may help delve into the ways in which low-fat but nutritionally empty foods such as potato chips and some crackers and cookies can lead to overeating and weight gain from the added calories in some people. The GI may be a useful tool for some diabetic individuals, since such individuals must control insulin response closely.

Energize for Exercise!

If you're an athlete and not aware that you need carbohydrates to fuel your workouts, then this is an exciting read for you! Carbohydrates, as will be discussed in the chapters devoted solely to pre-, during, and postexercise, are imperative to performance and recovery. The recommended daily carbohydrate allowance for athletes is about 2.3 to 3.2 grams per pound of body weight during periods of training, and even higher for those endurance athletes in season—it's closer to 3.2 to 4.5 grams per pound of body weight. Here are the carbohydrate needs for athletes:

For Training Days: 2.3 to 3.2 grams per pound of body weight
Body weight = 135 pounds
135 pounds × 2.3 = 310.5 grams
135 pounds × 3.2 = 432 grams

Carbohydrate range = 310.5–432 grams

For Endurance Athletes: 3.2 to 4.5 grams per pound of body weight
Body weight = 165 pounds
165 pounds × 3.2 = 528 grams
165 pounds × 4.5 = 742 grams

Carbohydrate range = 528–742 grams

Pre-, During, and Postexercise Carbs in Brief

If you're looking for details about what to eat before, during, or after your workout, you're probably going to flip to one of the chapters dedicated to the subject. For those who prefer to stick to the topic at hand, here's your exercise carbs chat in brief.

Pre-Exercise

Having carbohydrate-rich foods to help boost your blood glucose levels before exercise will help you exercise longer or at higher intensity compared to exercising on an empty stomach or with low blood sugar levels.

This pre-exercise meal or snack can be factored into the overall daily recommendations we gave you above. It's best to experiment with different types of carbohydrates to see which foods you tolerate best.

- Make sure the body is fueled at all times, especially with carbohydrate foods.
- Eat when you are hungry, as hunger is the best barometer of energy needs.
  - Eat five to six "mixed" meals/snacks that contain a combination of protein, carbohydrates, and fat per day.
  - Do not skip breakfast or go hungry between meals and snacks.

During Exercise

If you're exercising for over an hour, look to consume thirty to sixty grams of carbohydrate every hour, but bump that up if you are exercising for more than two to three hours to forty-five to ninety grams of the glucose-fructose blend in products such as PowerBar Gels or Performance Bars. Try sports drinks, gels, sports bars, fruit, crackers, or any other combination of easy-to-digest foods containing carbohydrates.

Recovery

We recommend eating a "recovery" meal or snack that contains proteins and carbohydrates within thirty minutes after physical activity. This will give you some extra fuel for muscle recovery and lean mass building. It also helps the body to begin building energy stores for the next training session or competition. If you've been engaging in physical activity for more than an hour, your glycogen stores have gone down and need replenishment.

- Within thirty minutes of exercise, aim to recover and start refueling your muscles for the next training session by eating 0.5 gram of carbohydrate per pound of body weight.
- If you plan on exercising again within the next twelve hours or so, repeat this intake every two hours for four to six hours after exercise, or until your regular meal schedule is resumed.
  - Recovery food should also contain protein (see the section on protein) for muscle repair.
  - Good recovery snacks include pasta with vegetables and lean protein, sandwiches, smoothies with protein powder, fruit and cheese, and many other "mixed" foods.

Close the Door on Carb Confusion

If you're not convinced that carbohydrates are a necessary, tasty component of your diet that provides energy for your active body, then we give up. Our last-ditch effort would be to remind you that without carbohydrates, your brain and body will eventually starve. The brain can only use carbohydrates for fuel, and the body requires carbohydrates for vital functions such as body temperature maintenance, blood circulation, and nutrient metabolism. In the absence of ample carbohydrates, the body will break down muscle and other lean mass for energy—leaving you weak and flabby. More specifically, in the short term this can lead to weakness, dizziness, higher perceived rates of exertion, and a number of other unfavorable conditions. In the long term it can lead to severe consequences such as electrolyte and acid-base imbalances and, potentially, kidney failure and heart arrhythmias. All sound terrible.

So please, enjoy a crusty, whole-grain baguette topped with fresh vegetables of all colors, lean turkey, and spicy mustard. Finish it off with a fresh fruit bowl with juicy strawberries, perfectly sweet grapes, and brightly colored cantaloupe!

4

Proteins: The Building Blocks

Protein 101

Everyone knows that they need proteins, but most think that they're just to build muscles. Proteins far exceed their role as musclemakers. Proteins are large, complex molecules in the cells of living things. They are an integral part of body structure, including muscle mass. Proteins differ greatly from carbohydrates and fats in chemical structure. Similar to carbohydrates and fats, proteins are comprised of carbon, hydrogen, and oxygen. But proteins also contain nitrogen. Nitrogen is found in amino acids, which are often referred to as the building blocks of proteins. Even amino acids can be further broken down, and the words "peptide," "protein folding," "genetic makeup," and "DNA" would eventually need to be discussed, so to keep it simple, we'll just keep in the back of our minds that proteins have a very complex and involved structure.

Amino Acids

Proteins come from both animal and vegetable sources. Animal sources include meat, fish, poultry, and dairy products. Vegetable sources include beans, nuts, and grains. While the focus of the discussion is proteins, it's not really proteins that our bodies utilize, it is the amino acid building blocks within proteins. There are twenty different amino acids in the protein-containing foods we eat, and the differing combinations of these amino acids make one protein different from another.

When you eat a protein-containing food, your digestive tract breaks the protein into its component amino acids, which are then absorbed and repackaged into the amino acid combinations that form the kinds of proteins you need. For example, when you consume a recovery beverage after you exercise that contains protein, the amino acids in that protein are released during digestion and absorbed. They are then repackaged into specific amino acid combinations to form the proteins you need to repair muscle tissue damaged during exercise and to build new lean tissue in response to your training.

More specifically, amino acids are molecules containing a central carbon atom attached to four other groups: a hydrogen atom, a side chain, an acid group, and an amine group (hence the name amino acid). The side chain of each amino acid is what differentiates one from another. There are only twenty amino acids, but these individual amino acids can be compared to letters of the alphabet. While there are only twenty-six letters, these letters can be combined to form countless words. These words, in turn, can be combined to create an endless amount of phrases. Similarly, while there are only twenty amino acids, combining these molecules to form various structures results in potentially a high number of unique types of proteins in living organisms. For example, the human body is estimated to form ten thousand to fifty thousand unique proteins.

Essential and Nonessential Amino Acids

Amino acids can be classified as either *essential* or *nonessential*. The two terms have nothing to do with the importance of an amino acid. Instead, they relate to whether the body can produce enough of it to meet physiological needs.

Essential amino acids are ones that the body cannot produce enough of and therefore must be obtained from food. Without enough essential amino acids in our body we lose our ability to manufacture whole proteins and other compounds vital to life.

On the flip side, nonessential amino acids can be made in sufficient quantities and therefore do not need to be consumed in the diet (if enough essential amino acids are present and adequate calories are consumed). Both essential and nonessential amino acids are depicted in the following table.

Essential Amino Acids	Nonessential Amino Acids
You must eat foods that have these	*Your body can make these*
Histidine	Alanine
Isoleucine	Arginine
Leucine	Asparagine
Lysine	Aspartic acid
Methionine	Cysteine
Phenylalanine	Glutamic acid
Threonine	Glutamine
Tryptophan	Glycine
Valine	Proline
	Serine
	Tyrosine

Protein and Amino Acid Supplements: Nice or Necessary?

Surely you have seen amino acid supplements on "health food" store shelves and even in your fitness club. With so many available, you must wonder, do I need one? If you are an athlete, the answer is an educated and confident . . . maybe.

First, though, note that many of these supplements are not telling the whole truth and nothing but the truth—some advertise themselves as the solution to your protein-poor diet, as a better-quality protein than what you could eat for lunch, or as a necessary supplement for optimal performance. We (and the science) say that these claims are unsubstantiated.

The other issue with protein supplements has more to do with amino acid supplements. Some contain only a few amino acids, and as we discussed, you need all of the essential amino acids to build protein. It's like if you were working on a puzzle and were given all the pieces that made up the sky, but not the ones for the landscape—you'd have only a partially made puzzle.

Value-Add?

Protein and amino acid supplements are typically based on food components. For example, they are dairy- (whey or casein), egg-, or soy-based. Because of this, in general, they have not been shown to provide any added or special benefit other than providing the proteins an active person may require. That said, there may be some benefit to whey protein that goes above and beyond its protein qualities.

Whey above the Rest

Research has begun to investigate whether whey protein has some additional benefit to athletes. Because it is thought to enter the bloodstream more easily than the other milk protein, casein, there may be support for choosing a whey protein if you're going to supplement. In addition, whey is rich in branched-chain amino acids that can be used for energy when glycogen is on the decline during long- duration activity—although we'd recommend taking in carbohydrate when your glycogen is running low. There is some evidence that it may help promote lean body mass increases, but the research is still mounting. We can say that if you choose to supplement with a protein, whey is the way . . . it will help you meet your protein needs, and the branched chain amino acid leucine is higher in whey protein, which may help drive muscle growth.

Determining Your Protein Supplement Needs

Regarding the question of whether an athlete requires a protein supplement, here are ways to determine if a protein supplement is a fit for you:

- What are my protein needs?
- Can I achieve this through my diet?
- Do I consume high-quality protein foods?
- Am I making proper choices if I am a vegetarian?
- How does this fit in my calorie needs?
- Have I confirmed this with a sports dietitian?

If you have answered no to some of these questions, do some research, read some labels, and according to the research, if you stay within your protein needs, you can safely enjoy a protein supplement.

You Complete Me

As you may have suspected, not all foods that are protein-containing have all of the amino acids. Some foods have all the essential amino acids; others do not. The superstars that contain all nine of the essential amino acids are considered high-quality, or complete, proteins. Many plant sources of protein do not contain all essential amino acids and therefore are considered low-quality protein foods and are even referred to as incomplete proteins. However, incomplete proteins—such as the proteins you might find in some grain products, lentils, and beans—are still good for you. You can take various incomplete proteins and combine them with other incomplete proteins to make a complete protein—or the proteins complement each other. Complementary proteins do not need to be eaten together; rather, think of it as a goal over the course of a day.

If you'd like to make a meal of complementary and consequently complete proteins, you can tap the old favorites red beans and rice, macaroni and cheese, peanut butter on whole-grain bread, spinach salad with pine nuts and almonds, and many other classic vegetarian dishes. It would appear that our ancestors, when faced with a lack of animal protein sources, had an uncanny knack for coupling plant sources to make high-powered proteins.

Protein sources differ in quality based on how digestible they are, but also on how well their specific amino acid combinations fit with what our bodies require to make protein. Thus, animal protein sources tend to be better-quality proteins than those from plants. But our diets often contain a mixture of protein sources from plant and/or animal sources, and this is usually more than adequate to ensure that all our amino acid needs are met. For the high-quality protein choices, those that provide all nine of the amino acids, here's a list to choose from. Remember to choose lean sources rather than high-fat options so that you get all the protein you need without the wasted calories from fat.

Complete (High-Quality) Proteins

Category	Food
Poultry	Chicken breast, boneless, skinless
	Turkey breast, white meat only
	Egg (whole)
	Egg white
	Egg substitute
Fish	Cod
	Flounder
	Haddock
	Halibut
	Trout
	Lox (smoked salmon)
	Tuna (fresh or canned in water)
	Salmon (fresh or canned)
	Catfish

Red meat/beef	Lean roast beef deli meat
	Select/Choice grade beef trimmed of fat
	Steaks of round, sirloin, and flank
	Roasts of rib, chuck, and rump
	Ground round or ground sirloin (drained)
Pork	Fresh or boiled ham, trimmed
	Canadian bacon
	Tenderloin
	Center loin chop
Dairy	Low-fat cottage cheese
	Fat-free cheeses
	Low-fat/2% milk-fat cheeses
	Skim milk
	2% milk
	Yogurt, light (artificially sweetened)

The Point of Protein

Why is protein so important, and what happens if I get too much or too little?

Protein has a myriad of functions, and neither athlete nor sedentary individual can live without protein. Proteins play a role in metabolism; they are a vital component of blood, the bones, and various hormones; they act as antibodies and therefore are important in maintaining immune function, good health, and fighting off diseases; and proteins help to maintain the body's acid-base balance and fluid status. The bottom line for the active person: the body avoids using protein for energy because it has too many other jobs that are more important.

How Much Do You Need?

Athletes consider protein the powerful macronutrient needed for muscle building. This is often a misnomer for the sofa lounger who believes that pounding beef jerky while watching TV will help him to bulk up. It depends on how you define "bulk up," but it won't help the body increase muscle mass if there isn't a stimulus . . . which is exercise. In fact, when protein is not used for a physiological function or to repair and rebuild after exercise, it is converted to and stored as fat. Figuring how much protein you need is a hotly debated issue. Look at the following table and find the range that best describes you:

Sedentary person	0.36–0.45 g per lb (0.8–1.0 g per kg)
Recreational exerciser	0.36–0.45 g per lb (0.8–1.0 g per kg)
Serious resistance athlete: early in training	0.68–0.77 g per lb (1.5–1.7 g per kg)
Serious resistance athlete: established training program	0.45–0.55 g per lb (1.0–1.2 g per kg)
Serious endurance athlete	0.55–0.73 g per lb (1.2–1.6 g per kg)
Teenage athlete	0.68–0.91 g per lb (1.5–2.0 g per kg)
Female athlete	15 percent lower than males

Active folks need more protein because they must take advantage of protein for muscle repair. Typically, protein deficiency and malnutrition are rare among athletes, but not impossible. If a person is very low in protein, it's most often related to his or her normal calorie intakes—if it's too low, his or her protein could be as well.

Poor Protein Intake

While in the United States protein deficiency is rare, it can occur. It is uncommon in athletes; it most often occurs in ill individuals or in individuals who are otherwise malnourished or restricting calorie intake. The effects of protein deficiency are immense due to the many roles protein plays in keeping our bodies functioning. We've seen protein-malnourished individuals who otherwise took in plenty of calories. On one occasion we worked with a young female who refused to eat anything but chips, pop, and snack cakes. Her parents were unwilling to recognize her eating issues and help provide simple solutions to help improve her overall diet. Consequently she arrived in a state of protein malnutrition, with thinning hair, pale skin, and a bulging belly from edema. Once she (or her parents) realized the need to eat properly and increase her protein intake, her malnutrition resolved.

Enough Is Enough!

On the opposite end of the spectrum is the individual who takes in too much protein. Usually this person is a male and usually an athlete trying to bulk up. There is speculation that high protein intake over time could increase the risk for kidney problems, bone loss, or heart disease. Here's the scoop.

Kidneys As far as increasing the risk for kidney disease, this is really important if you are at risk for kidney dysfunction, but it's not really an issue for most of the athletic population. The evidence is weak that eating a diet very high in protein causes kidney disease in healthy people. The concern is that there is evidence that a diet extremely high in protein increases protein breakdown and results in a by-product called urea, which is basically lost in urine. Therefore, athletes and individuals who choose to follow a diet high in protein should take care to consume adequate amounts of fluids to flush urea from the kidneys.

Bones There is controversy over whether diets high in protein cause bone loss. It was once thought that due to the high levels of certain amino acids (methionine and cysteine), calcium loss was increased. Because of the acid-base balance in the blood and since certain amino acids are acidic, calcium was pulled from the bones to act as a buffer. Currently the jury is out on this topic, and it is not clear that diets high in protein cause bone loss.

Heart The speculation that there is a link to heart disease is likely related to the types of protein foods eaten. If your favorite protein source is a greasy rack of ribs or a spicy buffalo chicken wing platter . . . well, you see the issue. If you're choosing lean meats, low- or no-fat dairy, and love skinless chicken and would rather pick fish, then your heart shouldn't be affected by your protein intake.

Protein for Exercise

Most active people we work with are conscious of their protein intake. They may think that they need more of it, they worry that without it they will lose muscle or not be able to gain it, or they think it provides them with additional energy for workouts. And more often than not, the response is to overload their diet with protein. Protein deficiencies are possible but rare. To add to the confusion, for years science has been trying to figure out exactly how much protein athletes require...and it's still debated today. But it is probably a moot point, since most Western diets provide more than the recommended amount. Proteins, like carbohydrates and fats, are also sources of calories or energy. However, protein plays a more important structural role in the body (e.g., as muscle) and therefore only about 1 to 5 percent of the protein you consume is used as an energy source. There are many options to explain and address the issue of protein with exercise. We think it would be easiest to break it down by the type of exercise.

Protein for Endurance Sports

As endurance athletes, you depend on your muscle mass to train for long-distance events. Since muscle is primarily made up of protein, it's understandable that athletes often question whether they're consuming enough protein, the right kinds of protein, and at the right time. And in fact, athletes do have greater needs for protein to meet the demands of endurance exercise, and timing of intake is important.

Most athletes meet their protein needs because of the sheer volume of food required to meet the energy demands of training. Instead of boosting protein intake further, athletes would be well served to consider the timing of protein intake in relation to training sessions. Training causes a breakdown in muscle tissue, and it provides a stimulus for muscle development. However, those processes can't proceed very effectively if amino acid building blocks aren't available for rebuilding or protein synthesis.

Endurance Exercise and Muscle Breakdown

It shouldn't come as a big surprise when you take a good look at the sinewy physique of elite endurance athletes: endurance exercise may increase muscle breakdown. We have to say "may," as it is very difficult to assess true protein turnover during aerobic activity. It's just tough to find the right tools to measure this in the lab.

This means that it is essential for endurance athletes to be mindful of their protein intake and time it right to help combat this breakdown by promoting synthesis. The jury is still out on whether protein should be consumed during exercise. There are a few studies that have found positive results when their subjects were given both carbohydrates and proteins

> *Energy to Burn Nutritionism:* Research has shown that a little less than four hours on the treadmill at 50 percent of your maximal effort can increase the rate of protein breakdown by 54 percent over rest.

during a long-duration activity. They found that there may be improvements in protein synthesis and muscle repair following the activity. What it comes down to is that recovery from endurance sport is the key (visit chapter 8 on optimal recovery if this has sparked your interest in what to do after your workout).

After an endurance exercise bout, the body is primed for protein synthesis for several hours. Some studies have shown that adding protein to a snack, meal, or beverage after a workout can help to increase glycogen storage if you haven't eaten enough carbohydrates for glycogen resynthesis.

There may be added benefits to consuming protein after a workout, however, that have more to do with repairing the muscles and improving protein synthesis. One study showed that by ingesting ten grams of protein with eight grams of carbohydrates (and three grams of fat) in a recovery beverage, there was an increase in protein-building.

When choosing your protein source after a workout, look to foods and sports nutrition products designed for recovery. These generally rely on protein powders as ingredients. Look at a label and you are likely to see whey and casein from milk, egg white powder from eggs, or soy protein from soybeans. These are all considered high-quality protein sources because of their digestibility and the fact that their patterns of component amino acids fit with what our bodies need.

FOODS AND SPORTS NUTRITION PRODUCTS FOR RECOVERY

Food	Serving Size	Protein Content (grams)
Chicken	3 oz	26
Fish	3 oz	22
Meat	3 oz	21
Milk	1 cup	8
Yogurt	1 cup	12
Cheese	1 oz	7
Cottage cheese	½ cup	14
Egg	1 whole	6
Peanut butter	1 T	4
Nuts	1 oz	6
Tofu	½ cup	20
PowerBar Performance Bars	1 bar	8–10
PowerBar Protein Plus Bars	1 bar	23
PowerBar Energize Bars	1 bar	6
PowerBar Recovery Beverage	16 fl oz	6
PowerBar Recovery Bar	1 bar	12

Branched-Chain Amino Acids

Of the amino acids discussed, three of them are termed "branched-chain" based on their structure. They are leucine, isoleucine, and valine. They are special because they can be used as an energy source for the muscles when needed. The use of these amino acids may come into play late in endurance exercise when glycogen stores are running low. About 25 percent of the protein in whole food sources is made up of these branched-chain amino acids. Despite their presence in food, supplement enthusiasts have investigated their role as an ergogenic aid.

Several studies have investigated the potential for performance improvements from branched-chain amino acids as a whole. Many have focused on their role in combating fatigue and fighting the effects of overtraining. Branched-chain amino acids present a theoretical advantage because they compete with tryptophan, an amino acid that is associated with mental fatigue (think about your post-Thanksgiving dinner nap; turkey has tryptophan). In theory, if you provide more of these branched chains, it should help to delay this fatigue. Thus far the role they have in fatigue hasn't been conclusive, according to the research.

There may be some relationship between branched chains and immune function, but this needs some work as well.

As a stand-alone branched chain, leucine has been investigated for its role in postexercise muscle synthesis. This research has shown some promising results for an additional benefit from protein with added leucine compared to the typical carbohydrate recovery intake.

BULKING UP

As you can imagine, building muscle is no easy task. It is quite a chore, requiring a stimulus and an intricate flow of cellular changes. Muscle growth will not occur if there is not a stimulus (i.e., physical activity or a heavy load, such as in resistance training). After stimulation, a number of events on the cellular level lead to muscle repair and subsequent growth. At the lowest level, muscles will grow when protein synthesis exceeds protein breakdown. Over an extended period of time, when this stimulus is consistently introduced, the muscles will hypertrophy (get bigger) and strength will increase. The extent to which the muscles will grow in size and strength depends on a variety of hormonal factors as well as on gender, age, and body size. At the heart of muscle growth, given a stimulus such as resistance training, you need protein to make the process successful.

The bottom line is that branched chains play a role in energy metabolism and may have some benefit to the athlete. Stay tuned as the research progresses.

Protein and Resistance Training

Given that muscles are made up of protein and that when we perform resistance exercise, the aim is to build muscle and subsequently strength, it doesn't take an exercise physiologist or a sports dietitian to figure out that eating protein is a good idea for weight lifters.

Unlike endurance exercise, there is less protein breakdown during strength work. A big *however* is that a resistance training session can lead to protein breakdown *after* a really strenuous session.

Because the potential for protein breakdown is higher after a resistance training session, attention to proper recovery is a must. It's simple: supply the body with essential amino acids and carbohydrates, and protein synthesis is enhanced. The result? You'll build more muscle and your proper recovery will lead to strength gains as you progress through your training regimen. Visit the chapter on optimal recovery for some postexercise meal ideas.

Energy to Burn Nutritionism: Researchers found that for three hours following a strenuous resistance training session, protein breakdown was 30 percent greater than at rest.

Green Eating

"A person does not need protein from meat and animal sources to be a successful athlete."
—*Carl Lewis, track legend*

Before delving into the discussion on vegetarian athletes, the definition of vegetarianism must be discussed. The practice of following a vegetarian diet often occurs on a continuum, with vegans being the strictest adherers to a diet void of animal products. Vegans typically consume only foods of plant origin. Therefore, they do not consume beef, fish, eggs, dairy, poultry, game, or any other animal products.

Some vegans follow this way of eating to the nth degree: avoiding any products hinting of animal use—from the seemingly benign

Energy to Burn Nutritionism: About four million Americans consider themselves vegetarians.

honey, multivitamins, and silk to the obvious leather boots, wool hats, and fur coats. Others who consider themselves vegetarians consume poultry and fish—although, we would say, that's not vegetarian eating. Still others avoid animal flesh but consume dairy products, eggs, and caviar.

WHICH TYPE OF VEGETARIAN ARE YOU?	
Type of Diet	Foods Consumed
Vegan	Plant-based foods only
Pesco-vegetarian	Vegetables, grains, nuts, legumes, fruit, seafood
Lacto-ovo-vegetarian	Vegetables, grains, nuts, legumes, fruit, eggs, dairy
Lacto-vegetarian	Vegetables, grains, nuts, legumes, fruit, dairy
Semi-vegetarian	Vegetables, grains, nuts, legumes, fruit, poultry, seafood, eggs, dairy

Why Go Veg?

The reasons for becoming a vegetarian or vegan are as varied as the types of diet. Some do it for ethical or religious reasons, others because of food safety and security, and yet others because of ecological or health benefits.

While it can be challenging for some to follow a vegetarian or vegan diet, the benefits of choosing this lifestyle are well known. Properly planned diets can be nutritionally dense and adequate and can reduce the risk of many chronic diseases. Vegetarians and vegans have been found to be at lower risk for obesity, heart disease, high blood pressure, type 2 diabetes, cancer, and more.

Not-So-Healthy Veggie Way

While a plant-based eating pattern can seem to be the utmost picture of health, if the diet is not well balanced and adequate in all macro- and micronutrients, vegetarians and vegans alike are at risk for nutrient deficiencies. It is well known that these specialized diets do not automatically mean that they are healthy. We know one lacto-ovo vegetarian who has now found that a breakfast of doughnuts and coffee, a lunch of grilled cheese, French fries, and pop, and a dinner of deep-fried falafel or pasta with cream sauce completely complies with his vegetarian choice. We've also come across young athletes who have chosen to follow a vegan diet for ethical reasons but who despise vegetables. As you can imagine, without the guidance of a dietitian, these young athletes are headed for severe deficiencies, compromised growth and performance, and a myriad of other problems.

In short, vegetarian and vegan diets can constitute a nutritional disaster if not properly planned.

Potential Veggie Pitfalls

Some of the most important nutrient deficiencies to be aware of include protein, calcium, vitamin D, vitamin B_{12}, omega-3 fatty acids, and iron. Luckily, many of these nutrients can be easily acquired from plant-based foods, fortified products, and the occasional dietary supplement.

Calcium Concern

Calcium is not present in dairy products alone. In fact, many lactose-intolerant individuals must acquire their calcium from alternate sources, which include, but are not limited to, calcium-fortified soy and rice milks, calcium-fortified juices, breads, cereals, and energy bars, seeds and nuts, and, of course, calcium supplements.

Because calcium and vitamin D are reliant on one another to function and often are in the same products, it makes sense that if at risk for a calcium deficiency, one is also at risk for a vitamin D deficiency. To combat this risk, it is likely that a vitamin D supplement is well warranted and close attention to the intake of vitamin D-fortified foods is necessary.

Be Aware of B_{12}

Consuming adequate amounts of vitamin B_{12}, or cobalamin, is one of the greatest nutritional challenges for vegans. Because vitamin B_{12} is most readily available from animal sources, vegetarians and vegans alike are at high risk for this nutrient deficiency, often referred to as pernicious anemia. Vitamin B_{12} assists in the formation of blood and, because it helps to maintain the sheath that coats nerve fibers, is essential for the healthy functioning of the nervous system. The consequences of a vitamin B_{12} deficiency are dire and include an increased risk of heart disease, diminished exercise tolerance, excessive fatigue, and other signs and symptoms.

While vitamin B_{12} is found in fortified products such as soy milk and cereals, many vegans tend to avoid these products. Vegans and individuals who avoid fortified foods must be diligent about taking a supplement. Some supplements and food items geared toward vegans claim to be potent sources of vitamin B_{12}. Here are some food items that are sources of B_{12}:

- Seaweed
- Algae
- Spirulina
- Nutritional yeast
- Fermented products such as tempeh and miso

While these items may contain B_{12}, it is not in the same form found in animal sources, which, unfortunately, is the active form of vitamin B_{12} that the body needs. The same can be said of beer; while it is a fermented plant product, don't bank on its supplying your daily dose of vitamin B_{12} no matter how much you are drinking. All in all, most solely plant-based sources of B_{12} are neither reliable nor very bioavailable; most likely a supplement is warranted.

Deficient in the Big Guns

Besides being at risk for *micro*nutrient deficiencies, vegetarians and vegans also can be at risk for a certain *macro*nutrient deficiency, the macronutrient being protein. When eating a properly balanced diet, the active vegetarian or vegan has no reason to experience protein malnutrition. One should be aware, however, that as stated before, not all proteins are equal and close attention should be paid to protein sources. By combining various plant sources throughout the day, essential amino acid needs can be met. For further thoughts on protein sources for vegetarians, refer to the following table.

VEGETARIAN SOURCES OF PROTEIN			
Food Item	Serving Size	Calories	Proteins (g)
Almonds	1 oz (22 almonds)	164	6
Barley	½ cup cooked	100	2
Black beans	½ cup cooked	113	8
Brown rice	½ cup cooked	108	3
Cheddar cheese	1 oz.	112	7
Chickpeas	½ cup cooked	143	6
Corn	½ cup cooked	82	3
Cottage cheese	½ cup	100	13
Egg	1 large egg	75	6
Grain-based burger (e.g., Gardenburger)	1 burger	100	5
Lentils	½ cup cooked	115	9

(continued)

(continued)

Food Item	Serving Size	Calories	Proteins (g)
Milk (skim)	1 cup	80	8
Pasta	½ cup cooked	87	4
Peanut butter	2 tablespoons	190	8
Peas	½ cup cooked	55	4
Soy "chicken" nuggets	4 nuggets	190	12
Soy "hot dog"	1 link	80	11
Soy milk (light, plain)	1 cup	70	6
Soy-based burger (e.g., Boca burger)	1 burger	90	14
String cheese	1 oz	80	8
Sunflower seeds	1 oz (142 seeds)	162	6
Tofu	½ cup cubes	94	10
Whole wheat bread	1 slice	70	3
Yogurt (low-fat, plain)	1 cup	155	13

5

Fats for Life: Fitting Fat into a Performance Diet

F-A-T IS A THREE-LETTER WORD, NOT FOUR. IF YOU ARE LIKE MANY ACTIVE people we talk to and counsel, you may believe that dietary fat isn't necessary healthful and that eating too much of it will turn your hard-earned muscular body into mush. Fat—whether it's on your middle or in your meal—is generally regarded as something to avoid. Despite lots of education about healthy fats and oils, dietary fat is still the number-one nutrient that people report they are trying to limit in their diet.

The right types of fats can improve your diet, boost the absorption of key nutrients, aid in postexercise recovery, and help maintain your sex drive. (Did we get your attention?) Fat may improve your performance, not hurt it.

Fat Facts

If you're confused about how much fat you should be eating and which are considered "good" or "bad," you're not alone. No matter how much you try to make sense of all the information out there about fat, deciding how to balance those fats in your diet to provide you with the energy and health benefits you need, without increasing the risk of heart disease, is a tough call.

Dietary fat is an essential nutrient, just like carbohydrates, proteins, or any vitamin or mineral. We need dietary fat for three main purposes:

1. To provide essential fatty acids that our body cannot produce;

2. To serve as a concentrated source of stored energy in the body; and

3. To digest and absorb fat-soluble nutrients and phytonutrients.

Without some fat in your diet, you can't transfer vitamins A, D, E, and K as well as many of the beneficial compounds found in fruits and veggies, such as carotenoids. Not essential to life, but also important, body fat helps to insulate your body when it's cold; it acts as a cushion around your organs to help protect them in contact sports or if you take a blow to your body. Ever wonder how your kidneys, heart, stomach, or liver would fare in any type of contact sport without having subcutaneous and visceral body fat to protect them? Or what diving into cold water would feel like without having some subcutaneous insulation?

Your body's stored fat, triglycerides are essentially like an unlimited fuel tank for you to tap into during exercise. Even lean adult athletes have 70,000 to 100,000 calories—about 120 hours of running at a marathon pace—stored in fat cells, muscles, and circulating in the bloodstream. That's about 700 to 800 miles worth of running, more than enough calories to fuel you from San Diego to San Francisco. Compare that to about 2,000 calories worth of carbs that the body can store when the muscles, liver, and blood are fully carbo-loaded—that's equal to about 90 minutes of marathon pace running. If the human body could use only fat for fuel, we would not have to worry about carbs, but since fat requires oxygen to be oxidized for fuel, it can supply the lion's share of energy for low-intensity exercise; but as oxygen becomes limited, carbohydrates become the major fuel source. Unless you want to exercise like a tortoise, you still need a high-carbohydrate diet to fuel your sports.

Numerous studies have been conducted to determine if athletes can "fat-load" their diets to maximize fat oxidation during exercise to try to spare the limited carbs the body has stored as glycogen. While an interesting concept, few of the studies found any beneficial effects of fat-loading or taking medium-chain triglycerides or showed any benefits in performance. However, it is now known that athletic training increases the body's ability to oxidize fat during exercise, so that the more fit athletes are, the more fatty acid they burn as fuel. Bottom line: to burn more fat as fuel, keep training.

Fat is the most energy-dense of the three macronutrients (proteins, fats, and carbohydrates), which is why sports nutritionists have typically recommended limiting fat for anyone trying to lose weight and why we use it to boost the calorie content with athletes who have a hard time meeting their caloric requirements. Each gram of fat provides 9 calories, more than double the calories you get from other nutrients. (Each teaspoon of oil or butter packs in 4.5 grams of fat or 40 calories.) By comparison, proteins and carbohydrates provide 4 calories per gram, while alcohol provides 7 calories per gram. However, more recent research suggests that when nuts and other unsaturated fats were included in a weight-loss diet, individuals were able to stick to the diet longer and felt more satisfied. Research also suggests that because fat is slow to digest, it aids in satiety, so that you feel fuller longer. For this same reason, dietary fat is generally not well tolerated in large amounts immediately before high-intensity exercise.

For athletes, fat requirements often take a backseat to the most important nutrients for performance, carbohydrates and proteins. As a general guideline, most athletes need to determine carbohydrate requirements first, proteins second; then the remainder of the calories should fill in as healthy fats.

The so-called healthy fats to focus on in your diet are monounsaturated or polyunsaturated. Diets rich in these types of fats, such as the Mediterranean-style diet, are linked with lower risk of many chronic diseases such as heart disease, diabetes, and certain cancers compared to diets high in carbohydrates and low in total fat or diet-rich in saturated fats and tans fats. In addition, several studies worldwide have found that there are health benefits to consuming diets richer in fats (albeit healthy unsaturated fats) compared to eating diets too rich in processed carbohydrates. However, these studies were conducted on sedentary individuals who didn't have the high carbohydrates that athletes have, so we're not recommending that you trade in your pasta for olive oil or go for peanut butter, not jelly. We are emphasizing that unsaturated fats aren't bad, and they appear to have health benefits that simple carbohydrates lack.

Studies over the past several decades have shown that the typical American diet—rich in saturated fats and omega-6 fatty acids and low in omega-3 fatty acids—may be contributing to chronic inflammation, central adiposity (increased belly fat), type 2 diabetes, and insulin resistance, among other health problems. Making changes to reduce saturated fats and increase unsaturated fats and omega-3s may help control inflammation and help reduce risk for all these health conditions. That brings us to getting to know the types of fats in our food and which ones you want to eat more of, and those you want to limit.

Saturated Fats vs. Unsaturated Fats

The more saturated a fat is, the more hydrogen molecules it has attached to its carbon chain and the more likely it is to clog arteries. Monounsaturated and polyunsaturated fats have fewer hydrogen and are less likely to trigger the process that creates plaque in arteries that impedes blood flow leading to cardiovascular disease, heart attack, and stroke.

Monounsaturated fat (monos) and polyunsaturated fats (polys) are considered the "good" fats. At the other end of the fat spectrum are saturated and trans fats, known to increase the risk for atherosclerosis and heart disease. When monos or polys are substituted for saturated fats or trans fats in the diet, they can lower total blood cholesterol and triglycerides (fats in the blood) and raise healthy, high-density lipoprotein cholesterol (HDL, the "good" cholesterol) levels in the blood. They also improve insulin sensitivity and help regulate blood pressure. Saturated fats and trans fats, on the other hand, are the "bad" fats. These fatty acids raise blood cholesterol levels and markers of inflammation, and are linked to excess belly fat. Excess saturated fat is associated with increased risk for heart disease, diabetes, and certain cancers.

The American College of Sports Medicine and other sports nutrition sources recommend 20 to 25 percent of calories from fat, the same as the Institute of Medicine's dietary fat guidelines for the general population. Other sports nutrition guidelines suggest a more individualized approach for determining dietary fat requirements based on caloric requirements and protein and carbohydrate needs. That means that for most active individuals, a dietary fat intake of 20 to 35 percent of total calories as fat, with an emphasis on more healthful unsaturated fats, is optimal. Dipping below 20 percent of calories from fat can increase your chances of disrupting your sex hormones. Low-fat diets in athletes have been associated with menstrual irregularities among female athletes and low testosterone levels among male athletes.

Making Fat Fit in a Performance Diet

Studies that have attempted to identify the dietary fat content of athletes' diets have found a wide range in percentage of calories from fat. Endurance runners and cyclists have been found to eat 27 to 35 percent of their calories from fat, and basketball players, rowers, and skiers got 30 to 40 percent of their calories from fat.

While fats are generally referred to as saturated, monounsaturated, and polyunsaturated, no dietary fat is 100 percent mono, poly, or saturated. Rather, they are combinations of all three in a wide variety of mixtures. However, one type generally dominates, and the fat will be labeled as either a saturated, polyunsaturated, or monounsaturated fat in the diet. Following are the fat basics on the major types of fat in our foods, and which to focus on for better performance.

Saturated Fat

What it is: The type of fat shown to clog arteries and lead to heart disease. A high intake also has been linked to an increased risk for some types of cancer. The harder a fat is at room temperature, the more saturated it is.

Where it comes from: Fatty meat, poultry, butter, cheese, cream, and whole milk; coconut, palm, and palm kernel oils; processed foods such as cookies, crackers, chips, and other baked goods. The top sources of saturated fat in the American diet are cheese, beef, and milk.

How much you should get: Aim for less than 10 percent of the day's calories from saturated fat. On a two-thousand-calorie-a-day diet, that would equal no more than twenty-two grams of saturated fat.

Trans Fat

What it is: A type of fat created when unsaturated fats are chemically altered (hydrogenated) to make them more solid. Trans fats are a component of partially hydrogenated oils, which are common ingredients in processed foods. They are used in food products to improve their taste and texture. Though they were originally thought to be a more healthful alternative to saturated fats, it's now known that trans fats act much like saturated fats, clogging arteries and increasing the risk for cardiovascular disease. Research also suggests that they can increase fat deposition around the abdomen, the location that poses the greatest health risk.

Where it comes from: Though an increasing number of food companies have removed trans fats from several products or have plans to remove and replace them with more healthful fats, many products still contain the unhealthy fats. French fries and doughnuts (unless they're specifically formulated to be trans-fat-free) often contain high amounts of trans fats. Small amounts of trans fats also are naturally in milk and nonskim dairy products, as well as in beef and butter. Research suggests, however, that only artificially produced trans fats pose a health risk. In fact, some of the trans fat in milk and beef occurs in the form of conjugated linoleic acid (CLA), which may actually be heart-healthy. Some studies suggest that CLA may reduce body fat, increase muscle mass, and could have anticancer benefits.

How much you should get: Some experts recommend limiting trans fats to less than 1 percent of daily calories (about one to two grams a day); others say zero artificial trans should be the goal. Foods labeled as "trans-free" are allowed, by labeling laws, to contain some trans fats (less than half a gram per serving). So eating several servings a day of so-called trans-fat-free foods could push you over the 1 percent limit. The Food and Drug Administration estimates that trans fat consumption is about six grams a day, far above what's recommended.

Monounsaturated Fat

What it is: Fat that falls between polyunsaturated and saturated fats. Studies show that diets that replace saturated with monounsaturated fats can lower LDLs and raise HDLs, while helping to control high blood pressure and possibly reducing the risk of developing type 2 diabetes. Monounsaturated fats are a core part of the Mediterranean Diet, which has been consistently linked with a reduced risk of cardiovascular disease. In the Mediterranean Diet, which is also characterized by a high intake of plant foods, little red meat, and moderate consumption of wine, olive oil provides more than half of fat calories. Olive oil also contains naturally occurring antioxidants called polyphenols that contribute to its health benefits; levels of polyphenols present vary depending on the type of olive used, the refining process, and how it is stored.

Where it comes from: Olives, canola, peanut oil, hazelnut oil, almond oil, sesame seeds, nuts, and avocados.

How much you should get: Ten to 15 percent of the day's total calories. A packaging symbol designed to help easily identify foods and beverages that belong in a Mediterranean Diet has been developed by Oldways Preservation Trust, a Boston-based nonprofit educational and advocacy organization. Called Med Mark, the postage-stamp-size symbol contains the image of an "amphora," a pottery jug used in Mediterranean cultures for centuries to store food and drink. Look for it on packages of healthful foods.

Polyunsaturated Fat

There are two major types: omega-6 and omega-3 polyunsaturated fats.

What it is: Polyunsaturated fats are unsaturated fats that have revealed themselves to be a healthy addition to the diet and the preferred choice over saturated and trans fat. Two of the polyunsaturated fats are essential to the diet: the omega-6 fatty acid, linoleic acid (LA); and the omega-3 fatty acid, α-linolenic acid (ALA). Both omega-6 and omega-3 fats have become the fats to focus on because they help maintain heart health and normal blood cholesterol levels.

Where it comes from: Omega-6s are found in vegetable oils, including safflower, sunflower, corn and soybean oils, including margarines, salad dressings, and mayonnaise made with these oils. It's also found in walnut and grapeseed oil. Omega-3s (see below) are in canola oil and in fatty fish such as salmon, sardines, albacore tuna, herring, mackerel, and rainbow trout. Omega-3s also are in grass-fed beef.

How much you should get: Up to 10 percent of the day's total calories, mostly as omega-3s (see omega-3s below). Because the typical American diet contains much more omega-6s than omega-3s, researchers worried that the imbalance could contribute to inflammation and blood clots and create an environment ripe for cancer growth. Subsequent studies have shown that the ratio isn't as important as once thought and therefore, we should be eating a variety of polyunsaturated fats and to replace saturated and trans fats.

Omega-3 Fat

What it is: A specific type of polyunsaturated fat that may help lower triglyceride levels in the blood, reduce the risk of developing Alzheimer's disease as you age, and reduce the inflammation associated with autoimmune diseases such as arthritis. Some research even suggests that it can be part of an effective therapy for depression. For athletes, its ability to tame inflammation also may apply to muscle damage during training, providing a potential advantage in recovery. The two most prominent omega-3 fats are docosahexaenoic acid (DHA) and eicosapentaenoic acid (EPA), which are used directly by the body. The form of omega-3 in plant foods is alpha-linolenic acid (ALA), which must first be converted by the body to EPA and DHA. The conversion is inefficient, so ALA is not as potent a source of omega-3s as EPA and DHA.

Where it comes from: The richest sources are fatty fish such as salmon, sardines, herring, albacore tuna, and rainbow trout. Most seafood provides 200 milligrams to 2,300 milligrams in a 3½-ounce serving. They are also in smaller amounts in walnuts and flaxseed oil.

How much you should get: There is no single official recommendation for how much omega-3s to take, but research suggests the following: If you're healthy, fatty fish at least twice a week.

Several studies and health organizations recommend more omega-3 fatty acids beyond what you will obtain from eating fatty fish twice a week. For example:

- Heart attack/heart disease: one gram a day from fish and/or supplements
- Athletes: one to two grams a day
- If you have high blood trizglycerides: two to four grams a day from supplements
- If you have rheumatoid arthritis: three grams a day from supplements

Omega-3 Supplements

Unless fish is a daily part of your diet, getting some of these higher daily amounts can be difficult, if not impossible. That's where omega-3 supplements come in. Are they safe? At least one study found that in some instances they may be safer than eating some fish, because they contain fewer toxins; the toxins are processed out during the manufacture of the supplements. Moreover, the type of fish typically used to produce supplements (anchovies, mackerel, menhaden, sardines) are less likely to accumulate mercury and other toxins, compared to larger fish.

Further reassurance of the safety of omega-3 supplements can be found in an analysis of omega-3 supplements by two organizations, Consumers Union and ConsumerLab.com. They found the fish oil supplements they tested to be free of mercury, PCBs, and dioxins. If you supplement, choose one with the highest level of DHA and EPA (they vary considerably), so you won't have to take a large number of pills each day. Another option is a flavored puddinglike supplement that provides 580 milligrams of EPA and DHA combined in each small packet.

Do not take omega-3 supplements if you take a blood-thinning drug such as Coumadin (unless you check with your doctor first), have had a stroke, or are scheduled for surgery.

Cholesterol

What it is: Not exactly a fat, cholesterol is a fatlike, waxy substance that travels through the bloodstream along with other fats. While it comes from the diet, the body also manufactures cholesterol, which is required to form cell membranes and some hormones. If it builds up in the blood, it can contribute to clogged arteries, increasing the risk of a heart attack.

Where it comes from: Cholesterol is found only in animal foods; plant foods are cholesterol-free. Shrimp, lobster, beef, chicken, eggs, and full-fat dairy products all contain cholesterol. Liver is exceptionally high in cholesterol. While eggs have been singled out as being the most commonly eaten concentrated source of cholesterol in the American diet, a large number of studies have demonstrated that eggs have little if any effect on blood cholesterol levels.

How much you should get: The American Heart Association recommends that healthy individuals limit their cholesterol intake to less than three hundred milligrams a day. People with heart disease should limit their intake to no more than two hundred milligrams a day. How well your body handles dietary cholesterol is in part genetically determined. Some people can eat double or triple the recommended amounts of cholesterol with no ill effects, while others can vigilantly restrict cholesterol and still find their blood cholesterol levels are too high and can be lowered only by medication.

Shopping for Healthy Fats

Stocking your kitchen with foods rich in healthy fats will help ensure that you're getting more of the unsaturated fats in your diet and limiting saturated fats and trans fats. However, to find saturated and trans fats lurking in packaged foods that might surprise you, use the guide below to understand fat-labeling regulations.

- *Fat-free*: less than 0.5 g fat/serving and reference amount set by the FDA
- *Low-fat*: 3 g or less fat/reference amount set by the FDA
- *Reduced or less fat*: 25 percent or less fat/serving than regular (full fat) product
- *Percent fat free*: Based on 100 g, when product meets the definition of low fat or is 100 percent fat free, claim can be made when a product meets the definition of fat-free and contains no added fat

You can also benefit from knowing what the following terms mean for meat, poultry, seafood, and game meats:

- *Lean*: less than 10 g fat, 4.5 g or less saturated fat, and less than 95 mg cholesterol/reference serving and per 100 g of the food
- *Extra-Lean*: less than 5 g fat, less than 2 g saturated fat and less than 95 mg cholesterol/reference serving and per 100 g of the food
- *Light*: Half the fat of comparable reference food. (If the food derives 50 percent or more of its calories from fat, the fat must be reduced by 50 percent.)

> **BUTTER VS. MARGARINE**
>
> The showdown between butter and margarine is as old as some of sport's best rivalries, such as the Yankees vs. the Red Sox or Michigan vs. Ohio State. The winner in our book is soft margarine. Here's why: butter is made from animal fat, which means it has saturated fat and cholesterol, whereas soft margarines are made from vegetable oils that are primarily unsaturated. And since most margarines are now free of trans fats, there's no reason to believe that butter is better.

Body Fat Energetics

There are different theories as to why excess body fat is associated with increased risk for many chronic diseases. Research suggests that fat tissue secretes hormones that increase inflammation. Inflammation can impact everything from cancer to kidney disease and heart disease. Fat tissue is also vascular, so extra pounds add additional strain on the heart, especially during workouts, without contributing to the body's ability to transport blood to muscles. In other words, it takes more heart muscle action to sustain healthy tissues when much of that tissue contains little additional blood vessels.

To gain body fat, you must consume more calories than you burn off. Period. Those calories can come from carbohydrates, proteins, fats, or alcohol. However, a key difference with fat is that it's the most efficient at being stored as body fat. If you consume more than a hundred calories a day of fat, ninety-eight of those calories will shuttle to your adipose storage in your belly or buns. Eat a hundred extra calories of carbs and seventy-five of those calories will be available to add to your love handles or chub rub. Enjoy a hundred extra calories of pure protein and sixty-five or so will be available to fill up your

> ### SHOULD I WORK OUT IN THE MORNING WITHOUT EATING TO LOSE FAT?
>
> A lot of athletes trying to lose a few pounds ask if they should skip breakfast and do their morning workout on an overnight fast. After sleeping for seven, eight, or nine hours, blood sugar levels are very low and fatty acids would be oxidized at low intensities. However, in practice, research shows that individuals who eat some carbohydrates before exercise are able to exercise harder and longer than those who skip a morning meal. So in essence, they burn more calories and wind up with a larger caloric deficit than those who skipped a meal, making eating before exercise the smarter option for overall body fat mobilization.

fat stores. This is because protein, carbs, and fats have different thermic effects, meaning that it takes more energy to metabolize protein than it does carbs, and fat requires virtually no energy to digest and absorb it.

To find how many grams of fat you need daily, locate the caloric intake closest to yours below, then find the corresponding grams of fat to equal 20 or 30 percent of those calories.

Calories per Day	20% Calories from Fat	30% Calories from Fat
1,500	33 g	50 g
2,000	44 g	67 g
2,500	56 g	83 g
3,000	67 g	100 g
3,500	78 g	117 g
4,000	89 g	133 g

It's estimated that Americans eat about seventy-five grams of fat per day. Here are the main food sources of that fat:

Food	Percent of Total Fat
Meat, fish, and poultry	30
Dairy products	13
Fats and oils	10
Grains and grain-based foods	8
Pastries and bakery foods	7
Eggs	3
Nuts	3

Chanmugam P, Guthrie JF, et al. Did fat intake in the United States really decline between 1989 to 1991 and 1994 to 1996? *JADA* 2003;103(7) 867–72.

Olive Oil

Olive oil is considered the oldest—and most popular—oil used worldwide. Supermarkets carry brands of imported oils from Spain (the world's largest producer), Italy, Greece, Tunisia, and other Mediterranean basin countries. All must adhere to standards set by the International Olive Oil Council. Olive oils are graded by taste, aroma, the amount of acid it contains and the processing it undergoes.

Next time you need to toss a salad, sauté vegetables, or bake, consider replacing colorless, flavorless corn and sunflower oils with the more healthful, vibrant olive oil.

Purchase smaller size bottles that are opaque (light can speed up oxidation of unsaturated fats) that you can use within three to four months. Always store in a cool, dark place for optimal taste. Here is a table of the types of olive oils available, why they're good, what they are, and how we can use them.

Type of Oil	Definition	Nutrition Bonus	Characteristics	Uses
Organic extra virgin	Contains less than 1 percent acidity; grown without use of chemicals; adheres to strict standards for aroma and flavor; least processed of all oils	Highest in polyphenols, tocopherols, and antioxidants	Rich in color, aroma, and flavor; may be fruity or nutty, depending on soil and types of olives	Dipping; salads; roasting vegetables; sautéing; will add olive oil tones to foods when cooking

Type of Oil	Definition	Nutrition Bonus	Characteristics	Uses
Extra virgin	Contains less than 1 percent acidity; must pass same taste and aroma standards as organic extra virgin; unrefined	Highest in polyphenols, tocopherols, and antioxidants	Rich in color, aroma, and flavor; may have fruit or nut tones, depending on olives used	Dipping bread; salads; sautéing; will add olive oil tones to foods in cooking
Fino (fine) virgin	Contains up to 2 percent acidity; contains a blend of extra virgin and virgin; may be refined	Processing results in a loss of some phyto-nutrients	Colorful, aromatic, and rich-tasting	Dipping bread; salads; will add olive oil tones to foods in cooking
Virgin	Contains up to 3.3 percent acidity; it is considered first press and unrefined oil, but oil may be heat-extracted	Moderate amounts of polyphenols, tochoperols, and antioxidants; same fatty acid profile	Less distinctive oil than the extra virgin or fino virgin oil	Cooking
Pure/light/ mild	Contains up to 3.3 percent acidity; made from virgin olive oil that is further refined to remove olive oil color and flavor; "light" or "mild" refers to color or flavor, not calories	Contains lower amounts of polyphenols, tochopherols, and antioxidants but has the same fatty acid profile	Pale yellow, no aroma; similar to corn or safflower oil	Cooking, baking

If you're like us, you suffer occasionally from olive oil overload. Thankfully, there's a whole new slew of specialty nut oils offering similar health benefits as olive oil.

All oils contain close to 40 calories and 4.5 grams fat per teaspoon. Like heart-healthy olive oil, these oils are rich in unsaturated fats, are low in the unhealthy saturated fats, and have no trans fats.

All the following oils contain significant amounts of vitamin E and beneficial phytonutrients that are found in the plants from which they are derived. Most of these oils are pricier than olive and other oils because they are hard to produce and therefore are produced in small quantities. To keep longer, they should be stored in a cool, dark place for up to six months; some need to be refrigerated after opening. Read package storage instructions for storage details.

Here's a look at some of the new artisan nut and fruit oils to hit gourmet markets:

Type of Oil	Nutrition Bonus	Characteristics	Uses
Extra virgin grapeseed oil	75 percent of oil is linoleic acid, an essential fatty acid; contains beneficial proanthocyanidins of grapes.	This green oil is nutty, buttery, and has winey accents.	Dipping bread; salad dressing; marinades for meat, fish, or poultry; finishing oil on top of grilled vegetables or fish
Walnut oil	Like flaxseeds, walnuts are rich in omega-3 fatty acids and trace minerals.	Amber oil that's smooth-tasting and has a nutty walnut flavor and aroma	Dipping bread; drizzle over cooked vegetables; top on fish or poultry; use as salad dressing
Avocado oil	Similar nutritional profile to olive oil; contains nutrients such as selenium and lutein and zeaxanthin present in avocados.	This vibrant green oil is full of nutty flavors and has the aroma of avocados.	Stable at high temps; can use this oil for baking, sautéing, and frying.
Hazelnut oil	Hazelnuts are one of the best sources of vitamin E and trace minerals.	Although pale in color, this oil packs a flavorful punch and has the aroma of roasted hazelnuts.	Salad dressings, sauces; combine with milder oils for cooking; can be used in baked goods.

6

Energize: Precompetition Nutrition

ONE OF THE GREATEST PERFORMANCE CHALLENGES, WHETHER YOU'RE heading out for a brisk walk, a three-mile jog, a studio cycling class, or an Ironman competition, is figuring out what and when to eat. When making this crucial decision, scan a list of questions in your head before your first bite.

- How will my food choices affect my performance?
- What will give me lasting energy?
- How much should I eat and when?
- What do I drink before exercise?

Let's break it down to answer these concerns and help you energize before you take your first step, pedal stroke, or dive. We'll review your needs before any exercise bout, so remember, precompetition may not be an organized event for you. It may be a hard-core workout at your local fitness center, a fabulous 5K you're doing for charity, or even your first long-distance triathlon. Whatever the day's challenge, energizing before exercise is essential.

Practice What You Eat

"I often see athletes (especially Ironman athletes) waiting until the last few days before their race to decide what their nutrition routine is going to be. My advice to them would be to experiment with different products and quantities in their training and less important races."

—Paul Fritsche, professional triathlete; most recent among his long distance accomplishments, second place in Ironman Wisconsin 2007

Nothing new on race day! Athletes and sports dietitians agree, do not try anything new on race day, from sneakers to snacks. Practice your precompetition intake as carefully and as mindfully as you train your body. Even if a race isn't in your future, trial and error will help you identify what works before your aerobics class. Your gut can be quite temperamental during physical challenges—even the research supports this—so practice what you eat to determine what sits well, keeps you energized, and makes you achieve your personal best.

Maximizing Stores: Carbo-Loading

Try to get a reservation at an Italian restaurant the night before a marathon and you'll be competing with racers to secure your party of five. Athletes recognize the importance of having adequate carbohydrates and load up on pasta and bread before an event. The rules of carbo-loading have evolved over the years, all with the same goal: to maximize carbohydrate (glycogen) stores. Studies revealed that not only is the body capable of storing more glycogen when fed more carbohydrates, but that this increase in stores can improve performance by 2 to 3 percent if exercising for more than ninety minutes.

> "The night before a race I like to have rice, grilled chicken, and a side salad with some fruit."
> —Peter Reid, three-time Ironman World Champion

It was once believed that proper carbo-loading required a period of depleting the body of glycogen followed by a few days of carb-supercompensation. This approach was characterized by three days of a diet of low carb, high fat and protein, and three days of high carbohydrate intake. Although glycogen stores were increased, restricting carbs for the first three days was difficult and even risky, increasing the potential for excessive fatigue, decreased immune function, and a poor mental state leading into race day.

More recent evidence has shown that three days of moderate carbohydrate intake (1.8 to 2.3 grams per pound of body weight) along with an exercise tapering period followed by at least one day of generous carb intake (3.6 to 4.5 grams per pound of body weight) can maximize carbohydrate stores for the big day.

CARBO-LOADING (3.6–4.5 G/LB OF BODY WEIGHT)		
Body Weight	3.6 g/lb Carb	4.5 g/lb Carb
130	468 g	585 g
140	504 g	630 g
150	540 g	675 g
160	576 g	720 g
170	612 g	765 g
180	648 g	810 g
190	684 g	855 g
200	720 g	900 g

How Will My Food Choices Affect My Performance?

It's likely you've heard the advice: gotta fill the tank before a road trip. Makes sense, right? If the dial is on empty, you are not going to get very far. The same goes for fueling your body before an exercise bout. Head out the door without any fuel and you're unlikely to make it to the bottom of the driveway.

There are two ways to consider how your food choices will affect your performance. Based on exercise studies, your performance can be measured by how hard you can push to get from point A to point B (exercise performance), and the length of time it takes you to exhaustion or fatigue (endurance capacity). What you eat before a workout can affect both of these.

Getting from Point A to Point B

Consider your workout: are you trying to last through an aerobics class, finish a hilly ride, or jog a 10K? Whatever the case, your intake before your bout of exercise can influence your ability to cross the finish line on your feet. A number of research studies have investigated this by giving some subjects a meal before an exercise trial compared to skipping the meal. The findings reveal that those who consume a meal, specifically one generous in carbohydrates, can do more work in a given time. Other studies have shown that carbohydrate supplementation up to four hours prior to an endurance activity can increase the duration of optimum exercise performance and intensity. This effect is enhanced when carbohydrates are consumed continuously during exercise (see chapter 7).

Time to Fatigue

Research trials that test how long it takes an individual to exhaust during an activity have shown a clear benefit from consuming a carb-rich precompetition meal. Not only are individuals able to last longer, but also a precompetition meal helps:

- maintain blood sugar (glucose) levels to stave off that dreaded drop in blood sugar;
- save stored carbohydrates (glycogen);
- improve performance.

Consider the results of this simple study protocol—subjects who skipped breakfast before the exercise trial bonked during their session. The study took seven cyclists and observed them as they cycled until they tired out. One group was given a hundred grams of carbohydrates three hours before exercise, while the other group exercised after an overnight fast. Exercise time was significantly longer for the athletes consuming breakfast in comparison with the athletes who exercised in the fasted state. Alongside the increased exercise time to fatigue, there were no negative effects on performance related to increased insulin and using fat as fuel after carbohydrate consumption.

Energizing for a Strength Workout

The stress of strength training and muscle building requires adequate calories. A range of twenty to twenty-three calories per pound per day is estimated to support these workouts. Shoot for an additional three thousand to four thousand extra calories per week when you're trying to maximize muscle growth. Of course, protein is an essential component for muscle growth and repair, but despite popular practices, an extreme level of protein is not necessary or warranted. Protein shouldn't be consumed at the expense of carbohydrates; carbs are especially important to those performing challenging resistance training workouts.

Prior to a strength workout, your needs are quite similar to your endurance needs, so our recommendations for pre-exercise nutrition apply to you as well. You want to have the best workout you can, so in addition to adequately hydrating, the preexercise meal should include carbs and protein (approximately fifty grams of carbs and fourteen grams of protein) one and a half to two hours before training.

What Will Give Me Lasting Energy?

Across the board—triathletes, weekend warriors, or soccer players—carbohydrates will give you that lasting energy. Not all carbs are the same, however, so it begs the question of which carbs are best. Researchers have investigated this question by comparing different types of carbohydrates and the effect they have on blood glucose as well as the insulin response. The research has mixed results; therefore it is not certain that it's worth paying attention to the glycemic index (GI) in your precompetition eating.

> "If it is an early morning race, I like to have eggs and toast with a glass of OJ and, of course, coffee! Oatmeal is also good prerace and I add nuts and fruit. If it is a race that requires another meal after breakfast, I have a peanut butter and jelly sandwich and fruit."
> —Katheryn Curi, Professional road cyclist who placed first at the 2005 National Road Race Championship, Park City, Utah

Because results vary from study to study, the American Dietetic Association (ADA) and the American College of Sports Medicine (ACSM) think that athletes should train with different GIs to determine the meal that works best.

> "[For a prerace meal] I have whole-grain oatmeal with pecans and dates or raisins, covered with vanilla yogurt—eaten three and a half to four hours before the race. I relish my prerace breakfast and thirty minutes before the start, I consume one gel."
> —Kevin Susco, PowerBar Team Elite Athlete

How Much Should I Eat and When?

Now we know that scheduling a meal before a workout is a must. Figuring out how much to eat and when is the next step. The timing of the meal is related to not only the need to fill the stores and provide energy for activity, but it is also important to consider how long the food will take to leave the stomach. It's a rare athlete who enjoys starting a workout with a full belly. Therefore, the experts agree that two hundred to three hundred grams of carbohydrates three to four hours before an event helps to refill glycogen stores, especially if this is following an overnight fast; increases endurance capacity; and extends the time to fatigue. The mean should include carbs and protein, and be relatively low in fat and fiber to improve the rate of digestion.

Here are some examples of meals containing 200 to 300 grams of carbohydrates:

Energizing at Breakfast

Sample 1

Four six-inch pancakes made from
  dry mix, prepared according
  to box
4 tbsp 100 percent maple syrup
1 cup fresh grapes
12 ounces fresh-squeezed orange juice

Totals

1,185 calories
208.5 g carbohydrates
23.5 g proteins
31 g fats

Sample 2

Homemade yogurt parfait
  1½ cups fresh pineapple
  ¼ cup raisins
  1 cup cereal
  6 ounces low-fat, light yogurt
1 medium low-fat blueberry muffin
16 ounces unsweetened apple juice

Totals

843 calories
204 g carbohydrates
18.6 g proteins
7 g fats

Sample 3

Peanut butter, banana, and
  honey on whole wheat
  2 slices whole wheat bread, toasted
  1 medium banana
  2 tbsp peanut butter
  2 tbsp honey
1 Powerbar Performance bar
8 ounces skim milk
16 ounces cranberry juice cocktail

Totals

1,225 calories
240 g carbohydrates
32.5 g proteins
21.6 g fats

Sample 4

    Cold cereal with fruit

        2 cups Rice Puffs cereal

        ½ cup apricots, dried and chopped

        8 ounces soy milk

    1 large apple

    1 medium banana-nut muffin

    12 ounces fresh-squeezed orange juice

Totals

    1,226 calories

    227 g carbohydrates

    26.7 g proteins

    18.8 g fats

Sample 5

    Honey oatmeal

        2 cups oatmeal (made with water)

        3 tbsp honey

    1 grapefruit

    2 slices whole-wheat bread, toasted

    2 tbsp fruit preserves

    8 ounces low-fat chocolate milk

Totals

    1,052 calories

    212 g carbohydrates

    28 g proteins

    10 g fats

Energizing Late-Day

Sample 1

    Simple pasta dish

        3 cups spaghetti

        6 ounces marinara sauce

        1 ounce Parmesan cheese

    2 slices white bread

    1 tbsp soft margarine

    1 cup broccoli, steamed

Totals

    1,124 calories

    200 g carbohydrates

    46 g proteins

    16.6 g fats

Sample 2

    Turkey and cheese sandwich

        2 slices whole-wheat bread

        1 slice low-fat American cheese

        3 ounces low-fat turkey luncheon
            meat

        1 tbsp fat-free honey mustard sauce

        1 leaf lettuce

Totals

    1,082 calories

    210 g carbohydrates

    42 g proteins

    13 g fats

Trail mix
    ¼ cup dried cranberries
    ¼ cup raisins
    ¼ cup low-fat granola
    1 ounce animal crackers
    1 ounce pretzels
1 cup grapes

Sample 3   *Totals*
    Long-grain rice and veggie teriyaki   1,154 calories
        1 cup long-grain white rice   225 g carbohydrates
        2 cups brown rice   36 g proteins
        1 cup Chinese mixed vegetables   11 g fats
        ½ cup teriyaki sauce
        1 cup diced pineapples
    12 ounces low-fat chocolate milk

Sample 4   *Totals*
    Peanut butter and jelly sandwich   1,243 calories
        2 slices whole-wheat bread, toasted   204 g carbohydrates
        2 tbsp fruit preserves   45 g proteins
        2 tbsp peanut butter   30 g fats
    2 ounces pretzels
    6 ounces low-fat, light yogurt
    12 ounces low-fat chocolate milk

Sample 5   *Totals*
    Couscous and veggies   1,168 calories
        2 cups couscous   268 g carbohydrates
        1 tbsp olive oil   32 g proteins
        1 cup mixed vegetables   19 g fats
    Banana berry parfait
        1 cup blueberries
        1 cup strawberries, sliced
        1 medium banana
        ½ cup low-fat granola
        6 ounces low-fat, light yogurt

Calculate your Preexercise Carbs

As the workout approaches, it is desirable to lower the amount of carbohydrates you take in to avoid stomach distress. Find your weight on the following chart to estimate the number of grams of carbohydrates to eat depending on the number of hours before your workout.

	1 Hour before Workout	2 Hours before Workout	3 Hours before Workout	4 Hours before Workout
Weight	*0.5 g/lb*	*0.9 g/lb*	*1.4 g/lb*	*1.8 g/lb*
120 lb	60 g	108 g	168 g	216 g
130 lb	65 g	117 g	182 g	234 g
140 lb	70 g	126 g	196 g	252 g
150 lb	75 g	135 g	210 g	270 g
160 lb	80 g	144 g	224 g	288 g
170 lb	85 g	153 g	238 g	306 g
180 lb	90 g	162 g	252 g	324 g
190 lb	95 g	171 g	266 g	342 g
200 lb	100 g	180 g	280 g	360 g

The Final Countdown

Within the hour before an event, some folks worried that eating may cause a spike and subsequent drop in blood glucose or block the body's ability to use fat as fuel. Despite this concern, research has shown that topping off the tank in the sixty minutes prior to working out actually improves performance. Experts agree that consuming carbs in the hour before the gun goes off will be beneficial.

> "I always have a PowerGel 20 minutes prior to any event."
> —Hollie Kenney, seventeen-time All-American and professional triathlete

With Sixty Minutes to Go . . .	Supplies	
PowerBar Performance Bar	230 calories	43 g carb
PowerBar Harvest Bar	240 calories	42 g carb
PowerBar Gel	110 calories	27 g carb
2 oz low-fat animal crackers	253 calories	42 g carb
2 oz dried apricots	282 calories	47 g carb

(continued)

(continued)

With Sixty Minutes to Go . . .	Supplies	
2 oz pretzels 2 tbsp hummus	263 calories	49 g carb
2 waffles 2 tbsp maple syrup	294 calories	56 g carb
Fruit smoothie 1 medium banana ½ cup diced pineapple ½ cup canned peaches in light syrup 8 oz skim milk	277 calories	63 g carb
1 cup macaroni ½ cup marinara sauce 1 oz mozzarella cheese	345 calories	40 g carb
1 cup Cheerios 2 tbsp raisins 4 oz skim milk 1 medium orange	282 calories	62 g carb

What Do I Drink before Exercise?

Staying hydrated is one of the most crucial and individualized goals of an active person. The American College of Sports Medicine (ACSM) recognizes the pronounced differences between individual sweat and electrolyte losses, variations among different types of activities, and environmental conditions. Therefore, staying in the hydration zone requires careful planning and practice. The aim of drinking before a workout is to help you stay in this hydration zone (euhydrated) and maintain normal electrolyte levels. Here is your precompetition hydration plan based on recommendations from the ACSM:

Four hours precompetition:

0.08 to 0.10 oz/lb body weight

Example: 150 lb individual = 12 to 15 oz

Two hours precompetition:

0.05 to 0.08 oz/lb body weight

Example: 150 lb individual = 7.5 to 12 oz

Try beverages with sodium or salted snacks to increase thirst and retain fluids.

Precompetition Intake Wrap-up

Let's put it all together and hit the pavement!

FOUR SAMPLE PLANS		
	Start in 3 to 4 Hours	**Start in 1 Hour**
Energize!	Peanut butter, banana, and honey on whole-wheat toast PowerBar Performance bar 8 ounces skim milk	PowerBar Gel 2 oz low-fat animal crackers
Hydrate!	0.08 to 0.10 oz fluid/lb body weight	0.05 to 0.08 oz/lb body weight
Energize!	Turkey and cheese sandwich Trail mix 1 cup grapes	2 oz dried apricots
Hydrate!	0.08 to 0.10 oz fluid/lb body weight	0.05 to 0.08 oz/lb body weight
Energize!	4 pancakes 4 tbsp 100% maple syrup 1 cup fresh grapes 12 ounces orange juice	PowerBar Performance Bar
Hydrate!	0.08 to 0.10 oz fluid/lb body weight	0.05 to 0.08 oz/lb body weight
Energize!	Homemade yogurt parfait 1 low-fat blueberry muffin 16 ounces apple juice	PowerBar Harvest Bar
Hydrate!	0.08 to 0.10 oz fluid/lb body weight	0.05 to 0.08 oz/lb body weight

Online Resource

At PowerBar.com you can register to get access to the latest in sports nutrition and training.

- **Connect** with other athletes around the globe
- Get your own **PowerBar profile** page featuring a unique URL
- Customize your personal site with **blogs, videos, and photos**
- Access leading-edge **sports nutrition** and **training tools**

- **Utilize interative tools to help you train and fuel for maximum effectiveness**

Two of the most popular features on the site include:

PowerCoach PowerCoach is the first global nutrition-based online customizable training program. By offering users personalized nutrition and training from top athletes and sports nutritionists, PowerCoach can help improve your performance.

Ironman 29-week Training IronmanPower.com offers the latest nutrition as well as interactive tools to help train for the grueling Ironman event. The 29-week Ironman training and nutrition guide also includes tools like RouteFinder and personalized widgets to post on your favorite social networking site.

7

On the Go: What to Eat and Drink When Active

The first nine miles of the run went pretty well, but some-where around mile ten, I started to feel nauseated, and then threw up at mile thirteenish and again at mile seventeen and at mile eighteen. I couldn't hold anything down—even while walking—until mile twenty-three. At that point, I had decided I was going to die if I didn't drink and die if I did. I crossed the finish line some fifty minutes later.

—*David Pollard, 2008 Ironman Arizona competitor*

I didn't eat or drink enough . . . I'm on the rivet in the lead break for most of the day and could barely think about taking my hands off the handlebars. On the last climb, I'm feeling my VMO muscles cramp, then it really hits me, and I can barely turn the cranks over.

—*Craig Upton, Cat I road cyclist*

LIKE THE ABC SPORTS TAGLINE "THE THRILL OF VICTORY . . . AND THE agony of defeat," there's something about watching an athlete bonk, choke, or go from bad to worse in seconds that grabs our attention. Research shows that more often than we ever thought, sports nutrition plays a role in an athlete's demise.

Generally, the longer the event, the more important nutrition during exercise matters, but more recent research shows that nutrition *and* proper hydration during exercise improve just about everyone's performance. Decades of research show how endurance athletes need to stay hydrated and have carbs to avoid "hitting the wall," but newer studies show that athletes competing in short-duration, high-intensity sports such as skiing, ball sports, and tennis as well as precision athletes such as golfers and race car drivers need to pay attention to their hydration and energy requirements during their events to optimize their game.

In our years of working with athletes, we've seen or heard about countless races lost, Olympic medals missed, and failure to reach one's potential from overlooking hydration and nutrition during exercise.

In previous chapters, we've covered what constitutes a performance diet, what you need to eat when you're not working out, and day-of-event nutrition strategies. Now it's time to focus on what you should (and shouldn't) be eating and drinking while you exercise. Basically, we'll provide you with all the information to help bonk-proof your body. What you eat and drink during exercise can supply the hydration and carbohydrates to fuel your muscles to help you be your best.

This chapter will provide the guidelines for endurance athletes, nonendurance athletes, and those who may have multiple exercise sessions in one day.

Regardless of the sport in which you participate, there are considerations that apply to all athletes, including:

- time(s) of day of your event;
- duration;
- intensity level;
- level of anxiety or nervousness;
- environmental conditions (heat, wind, cold, precipitation);
- what's available to eat/drink during the event;
- number of aid stations or access to fluids/food; and
- your taste, texture, and flavor preferences in those conditions.

There are two primary goals of drinking and eating during exercise: to avoid dehydration, and to supply a steady supply of highly combustible carbohydrates for anyone exercising for an hour at one time, or more or multiple times in one day.

First, let's focus on optimal hydration as it is the most important factor for during exercise nutrition, and it has the biggest consequences if ignored.

Optimal Hydration during Exercise

Check out this amazing story from Josh Cox, elite marathon runner and youngest qualifier for the 2000 U.S. Olympic marathon trials:

It was early summer 2004. I was training from my home in Murrieta, California, about sixty miles northeast of downtown San Diego. This particular training cycle was sandwiched between my seventh-place finish at the Olympic marathon trials and my U.S. Team appearance at the world half marathon championships in India.

As a marathon runner my training regimen calls for both morning and evening sessions. The breakdown is typically ten to fifteen miles in the morning and six to ten in the evening. Sixty to ninety minutes in the morning, thirty to sixty in the afternoon with core work, lifting, stretching, writing, and resting supplement the remainder of the day.

Once every ten days or so the schedule calls for a twenty-five-to-thirty-miler where the idea isn't to run it as fast as you can but rather to maintain a good effort and cover the distance. So on this day I woke up just before ten, drank my coffee, read the paper, and got ready for the run. Just before noon I walked my coffee out of the comfort of my sixty-nine-degree house onto my porch to check the conditions. When you live twenty miles inland in Southern California, you never know when the warm winds from the Santa Ana Mountains will blow through. When they do, it feels like God left His hair dryer on. As I stood on my porch, I surmised His hair dryer was not only on—but He also left it on high.

I considered delaying the run until the late afternoon, but not being one to let a perfectly good caffeine buzz go to waste, I figured I would brave the high noon elements. Most days I drive the course and stash bottles filled with sports drinks every three or four miles, but out on my porch I have a thought . . . no, an epiphany. I can do this long run without any fluid support.

Now, I realize most humans would never consider, much less attempt, running more than twenty miles without fluids, but as a professional athlete I am, at times, delusional and lose touch with my mortality. Now, through therapy, I can admit that I have a bit of a superhero complex. I mean, I can string together a series of sub-four-forty miles, I've run fifty-mile races, I've run twenty-five miles with no fluids before—I can do it again.

So I set out in my shorts, shoes, and MP3 player, and despite the heat, I'm in the zone. Any athlete will tell you that every so often the stars align and everything comes together. On those days when you feel you can do anything; on those days you feel like a superhero.

On long run days I like to run out-and-back courses. This way if I were to get any funny ideas about cutting the run short, I can't. There's only one way out and one way back. This particular course was pretty desolate. It travels along Winchester Road and heads out toward a town called Hemet. I don't know much about Hemet other than that it smells like cows and serves as a cut-through on the way to Palm Springs.

So I was hammering along the dirt shoulder and passed ten miles in less than fifty-three minutes—that's right around a five-minute pace for the last five. I reached the twelve-and-a half-mile mark—the twenty-five-mile turnaround—but things were still going pretty well so I figured I'd run the full fifteen and get in thirty for the day. I reached fifteen in under one twenty-three—that's right at a six-minute pace for the last five. I'm slowing, but still feeling good.

The next five passed without incident, but I began to feel the effects of the heat. I switched my music back to the slow mix and slowed the pace in an attempt to preserve the effort.

Then things started going badly. Anyone who has run beyond twenty miles in the heat will tell you, things can go from good, to bad, to worse, to you're totally screwed in about the time it took you to read this sentence. Pardon the juxtaposition phrase but things tend to snowball in the heat.

I'd guess I was still running seven-minute miles or so but I was slowing by the second; pretty soon this was going to be a death march. My mouth was dry, my throat was dry, I couldn't spit, I was no longer sweating, and I was dehydrated—the white, pasty sweat on my chest and arms told me so.

I'm no superhero—I'm an idiot. Only a fool would try to run thirty miles in horrible heat with no water. Reality: I am susceptible to the same natural laws as everyone else. People need water. Runners need even more.

I kept running—using the term loosely now—and began licking my arm. And before you laugh or vomit, don't knock it till you try it. Once, in college, I separated myself from the group on a run in the Blue Ridge Mountains and proceeded to get myself thoroughly lost for six hours, and after thirty-five miles of running resorted to drinking the highly sought-after delicacy of puddle de la mud. Best mud I ever tasted; granted, the only mud I've tasted, but good mud nonetheless; comparatively speaking, the salt and sweat tasted like surf and turf. You don't know what disgusting things you're capable of until you find yourself fighting to survive.

So there I was, the wheels were coming off, I can't stop because I know how hard it will be to start again, there isn't anything around, and to top it all off, in my many years of training I've never failed to reach my destination. I can't stop now. My running rule, and life rule, for that matter, is "Keep moving forward."

So I start to pray. "Lord, I'm really stupid. I'm in a lot of trouble here. I still have a long way to go and if I don't get some water I won't make it. So if you could hook me up, I'd appreciate it. Maybe you can have someone pull over for some directions and give me water."

I run around fifty times a month, which, over the course of the year, makes for roughly six hundred times I lace up the shoes and pound the pavement. Out of those six hundred runs a passerby will stop to ask me for directions five times, perhaps six if it's a leap year.

So I continued running and for the next minute continued offering up all sorts of ways He could deliver me some water. "Someone could get a flat, or one of my friends could drive by, a crazed fan could stop for an autograph, a girl could stop for my number." They were all solid suggestions and things that had happened in the past. You know, just in case God was short on ideas.

A minute later a blue midsize car pulls over onto the dirt. My water has arrived.

The car stopped about thirty feet in front of me. I stopped the music and slowed to a stop. A lady exited the car and walked toward me. I don't totally understand the physiology of what happened next, but when I stopped I felt a cold rush to my head and I lost my balance and fell forward. Fortunately I managed to get my hands out onto the dirt and saved myself from falling. Being an egomaniac too proud to admit he had fallen over, naturally I played it off like I was doing a hamstring stretch. I stayed bent for a few seconds and waited until my equilibrium returned. The woman's feet appeared in front of me and I rose out of my jackknife.

"Are you okay?" she asked me.

"Oh, yeah, just stretching."

I should have said no and begged her for a ride, but superheroes don't need rides.

"Okay, well, do you know how to get to Pechanga?"

"What you want to do is head back that way to 15 south and it's the second exit. You'll see the signs from there."

"Thanks!"

She started walking back to her car.

"Um, miss? Do you have any water with you?"

"I'll check."

She walked to her car and returned with a bottle of Arrowhead water.

"I took a sip," she says, "but you can have it since you gave us directions."

"Thanks, much appreciated."

After that I made it home. I stepped on the scale. I had lost more than ten *pounds*. Things nearly went very, very wrong. The news that night said the inland area temperatures topped more than a hundred.

You'd think that an athlete at the highest level of his sport would know better, right? Well, unfortunately, Josh's story is somewhat common among athletes—and in fact, sometimes the fit athletes are the ones who feel the most invincible and are likely to forgo appropriate planning for hydration and nutrition during exercise.

As simple as it may seem, H_2O is the elixir of life and is required for every cell and virtually everything our body needs to do—from digesting that banana you just ate to blinking your eye or flexing your bicep. That's why we can survive for weeks (maybe even months) without food, but without water, we will die in days.

Optimal hydration is key for athletes because sweat evaporation off our skin is our major defense against heat-related illnesses. As sweat evaporates off skin, it cools the body. When you exercise in hotter weather, the body will increase sweat production to help keep your core temperature from rising. Wiping yourself dry during exercise reduces the body's natural thermoregulation. So, too, does high humidity. If ambient air's moisture content rises to that of wet skin, evaporation is impaired and sweat will just bead up and roll off your skin. This is why hot, humid conditions are the most difficult for athletes to keep and stay hydrated in to avoid heat illness.

Losing just 2 percent of your body fluids (just 3 pounds lost during exercise for a 150-pound athlete) can compromise your athletic performance and pose health risks. To put fluid into perspective, when you run out of carbohydrates during exercise, you bonk, but other than bruising your ego, you'll be fine. However, if you get severely dehydrated and drive up your core temperature, you can die. Decades of research has shown that dehydration reduces muscle strength, power, speed, stamina, and cognitive function; at the same time, it increases risk of injury.

Most athletes will replace only 30 to 70 percent of the total fluid they lose during exercise, according to the Australian Institute of Sport. Most active individuals will lose one to two liters of fluid per hour during strenuous exercise, and there have been reports of losses of three to four liters per hour in very hot and humid conditions among high-level athletes. Men generally sweat more due to their larger body mass and high metabolic rates compared to women. Not only do sweat losses vary greatly; so, too, does the electrolyte composition of the sweat produced by the two million to four million sweat glands in your body.

For example, among pro football players, researchers found a tenfold difference in the amount of sodium lost in athletes' sweat, indicating that some of us are just "heavy sweaters" and others are not. Sodium is the primary electrolyte lost in sweat, and is the electrolyte that needs to be replenished during exercise. Studies do not indicate that chloride, potassium, or magnesium need to be replenished during exercise to enhance performance, even among endurance and ultraendurance athletes.

Making optimal hydration even more difficult is the fact that everyone has his or her unique sweat rate, and two athletes of the same size exercising at the same intensity could have very different sweat losses. As a result, numerous sports medicine authorities, including the American College of Sports Medicine, the American Dietetic Association, and the National Athletic Trainers Association, now recommend individualized hydration analysis so athletes can tailor their fluid intakes to sweat rates. Following are some of the basic hydration guidelines these organizations recommend.

Basic Hydration Guidelines during Exercise

- Six to eight ounces every fifteen to twenty minutes, or
- Eighteen to thirty-two ounces per hour

As you can see, this wide range in fluid ounce intake isn't that practical for most of us, as it's too general. To tailor hydration recommendations for your needs, it's necessary to calculate your optimal hydration zone. The only practical way to do this is to test your sweat rate at an exercise intensity and in climate conditions similar to those you expect to encounter in your training or upcoming event. We also recommend testing yourself every month or so during your key training phases to fine-tune your hydration plan for whatever conditions (and your fitness level) you may be training or competing in. A handy sweat rate calculator can be found at PowerBar.com.

Also, athletes need to keep tabs on their hydration status whenever they're in training or in the competition phase. To do this, weigh yourself most days of the week to ensure that you are fully hydrated after workouts. If you wake up lighter than normal, it's likely due to dehydration, so drink twenty to twenty-four ounces of fluid for each pound (sixteen ounces) you are down on the scale. In addition, check your urine: if it's light in color or colorless, you're hydrated; anything darker than lemonade and you need to drink more. If the color is like apple juice or cola, you could be damaging your kidneys.

To speed the stomach's ability to handle liquids, it is best to always have some fluid or food in the stomach. For example, start with seven to ten ounces of water or sports drinks ten to twenty minutes before exercise to slightly distend the stomach so it promotes more rapid emptying of fluids. Practice this with varying amounts of fluid to see the amount that works best for you preexercise to keep you hydrated. Of course, drinking beverages that you like the taste of and that work for you is important. Water and sports drinks are the preferred fluids for most athletes, as beverages that have too high a sugar content actually slow stomach emptying.

Sweat Rate Calculator

Since sweat rates vary due to sex, fitness level, body weight, and ambient temperature and humidity, the only way to get a good handle on how much you sweat in various conditions is to weigh yourself before and after workouts to assess your losses. Here's how to figure your optimal hydration zone:

Body weight × .02 equals pounds that you cannot exceed lost in sweat. For example, if Jane weighs 125 pounds:

125 × 2% body weight = 2.5 pounds

125 – 2.5 pounds = 122.5

Jane's hydration zone is 122.5 to 125 pounds. She wants to calculate her sweat rate so she knows how much fluid per hour she needs to drink to keep from losing more than 2.5 pounds in fluid losses during exercise.

Calculate Your Hourly Sweat Rate

1. Weigh yourself prior to a one-hour workout.
2. Calculate in fluid ounces how much water or other fluids you drink during the one-hour workout.
3. Weigh yourself after the workout.

Calculate the sum of your postworkout weight lost plus the fluid ounces drunk; if that is lower than your start weight, you need to increase your fluid intake by the deficit to match that intake.

Example: Jane, who weighs 125 pounds, runs for 1 hour and drinks 4 ounces during the run. She weighs 124.5 pounds at the end of her run.

8 ounces lost in sweat + 4 ounces = 12 ounces/hour sweat rate

Keeping Up with Your Sweat Rate

Knowing your sweat rate is the first part of the equation, but the other half of the equation involves setting up strategies to *actually* drink all that fluid. Most athletes find it difficult and uncomfortable to consume fluids at a volume that matches their sweat rate. The Australian Institute of Sport has found that athletes generally drink only 30 to 70 percent of their sweat rate, which is why dehydration is so common. If that is the case for you, remember that your hydration zone is losing no more than 2 percent of your preexercise body weight due to fluid loss during exercise. So you don't need to exactly match your sweat rate. Instead, you need to make sure you don't drop out of your zone while you are exercising.

Example: Tom weighs himself before a run and is 155 pounds. He drinks 6 ounces during his 1-hour run and weighs 154.5 pounds after the run.

Preexercise weight = 155 pounds

Postexercise weight = 154.5 pounds

Fluid ounces drunk = 6 ounces

Total fluid loss = 14 ounces (8 ounces lost + 6 ounces)

Using the calculation for hourly sweat rate, Tom's hydration zone would be 152 to 155 pounds.

Tom's results indicate that he remained within his hydration zone during the test. However, if Tom plans on competing in a marathon or Ironman, that 14-ounce deficit per hour could easily add up to an energy-zapping deficit in about 3½ hours.

Tom should repeat the test in a few weeks, and try to drink 12 ounces of fluid (6 ounces every 30 minutes) in the hour trial to see if he can more closely match his fluid losses.

Sports Drinks versus Water?

As a general rule, most sports nutritionists recommend fluid and electrolyte replacement (aka sports drinks) with 4 to 8 percent carbohydrate concentration that contains sodium, the primary electrolyte lost in sweat. Sports drinks not only deliver fluid to ward off dehydration, they also provide carbohydrates and electrolytes, mainly sodium, the primary electrolyte lost in sweat, in a rapidly absorbable formulation. A sports drink within the recommended carbohydrate concentration and sodium will be absorbed in the GI tract faster than plain water.

The addition of sodium will also help continue to "drive" your thirst so that you continue to drink. We also recommend sports drinks that use a combination of glucose, maltodextrin (glucose polymers), sucrose, and fructose, generally with more of the glucose and sucrose and less of the fructose. Mounting research suggests that glucose, sucrose, maltose, and maltodextrins are oxidized at higher rates than fructose, which is digested slowly by the small intestine and must be converted by the liver to glucose, then released back in the bloodstream before the muscle can use it as energy. A solution containing a combination of glucose and fructose, however, was shown to increase total carbohydrate oxidation rate by 20 to 40 percent or even more over the same beverage and caloric intake but sweetened with glucose only. In addition, studies have reported that consumption of energy drinks and products that provide some fructose may be better tolerated (possibly fewer GI complaints) than those without fructose. Multiple carbohydrate transport mechanisms are proposed as the reason for the enhanced rate at which the body can burn carbs. Use the chart on pages 114 and 115 to compare popular fluid and electrolyte replacement drinks.

In some cases, athletes prefer plain water, and that can be fine as well. If you drink water only, the concern is to get more carbohydrates and sodium through sports nutrition products and real food to meet the hourly recommendations.

Weight-conscious athletes may benefit from using lower-calorie fluid electrolyte beverages, which provide lower amounts of calories and carbohydrates with sodium to enhance hydration.

How to Meet Your Fluid Needs

There are many strategies athletes employ to ensure that they are well hydrated. Here are ten of our favorites for normal, everyday hydration:

1. Set your wristwatch to beep every fifteen minutes to remind you to drink.
2. Plan your exercise route based on where you have water stops or where you have placed sports drinks beforehand.
3. Experiment with hydration packs such as those from CamelBak or Ultimate Direction to see which works best for you.
4. Keep reusable sports bottles filled with your favorite sports drink in your gym bags, locker, and on the bench to encourage drinking.
5. In supported events, know ahead of time which fluid stations you will use and how much you need to drink, and stick to your plan.
6. Match your fluids to the conditions. Hotter days may require fruitier, more bitter flavors, whereas other flavors are best for cooler temperatures.
7. Keep a water bottle on your desk at work and drink from it frequently during the day. Set a goal for the amount of fluid you should drink daily, and reward yourself when you achieve that goal.
8. Dilute fruit juices to maximize your hydration and minimize their empty calories.
9. Drink before you're thirsty. Generally, by the time your brain signals thirsty, you are slightly dehydrated.
10. Drink early and drink often. It's easier to keep up with your hydration than getting behind it and having to play catch-up.

Water on the Brain?

While the vast majority of athletes suffer from dehydration, a growing number of athletes drink too much water during endurance exercise and develop a life-threatening condition when their blood sodium levels drop below normal levels. Low blood sodium levels disrupt the normal osmotic balance across the blood-brain barrier and cause water to seep into the brain, leading to cerebral edema (brain swelling). That's a bad thing.

Symptoms may begin with headache, confusion, malaise, nausea, and cramps—all similar to signs of dehydration—making some mistake hyponatremia with dehydration. Two telltale signs of hyponatremia are weight gain and puffiness. Athletes will notice that jewelry or even elastic in their apparel will feel tighter. If it is not corrected and gets worse, serious outcomes such as seizure, coma, and death from brainstem rupture can occur.

Hyponatremia tends to be more common among slower endurance athletes (e.g., marathon runners, cyclists, and triathletes) who are out on courses for many hours and drinking excessive amounts of water, as opposed to sodium-containing sports drinks. It is also up to three times more likely among female athletes than male (smaller body size appears to be key, not so much gender), and misuse of nonsteroidal anti-inflammatory medications may increase risk. Studies have found that 10 percent or more of Ironman and marathon finishers have some degree of hyponatremia (most not severe), and the number-one sign is weight gain. In case we didn't convince you earlier that sports drinks are best, hyponatremia is the last straw that should hopefully make you a convert.

Are You a Salty Sweater?

To determine if you have a high concentration of sodium in your sweat, answer the following questions. If you answer yes to two of the three, you are a salty sweater and require more sodium before, during, and after exercise to help stay hydrated.

- My clothes are usually caked in white sweat after a strenuous workout.
- I have salt visibly caked around my hairline and face.
- My eyes burn when I'm working out hard and really sweating.

The Eight × Eight Myth: How Much Fluid Do You Really Need?

Everyone has heard that we need to drink eight eight-ounce glasses of water each day, but as you will see, that's another one of those old wives' tales that's been passed along for generations.

The National Academy of Sciences report on the dietary reference intake for average *sedentary* adults is equal to the following:

Women: 91 ounces per day total (fluids + foods)/73 ounces from fluids only = twelve 8-ounce glasses of fluid per day

Men: 125 ounces per day total (fluids + foods)/100 ounces from fluids only = twelve 8-ounce glasses of fluid per day

In a typical diet, 80 percent of our fluid intake comes from foods and the other 20 percent from water-rich foods such as fruits, vegetables, and grains. This same report also gave the okay for all beverages counting for daily fluid intake—including caffeinated beverages and alcoholic beverages.

Signs of Heat Illness

Heat Stroke

Inadequate fluid intake during exercise can greatly increase your odds of heat stroke, the most serious of heat illnesses. Signs include:

- headache, dizziness;
- nausea, vomiting;
- weakness, loss of power;
- irritability;
- inability to concentrate, confusion;
- high body temperature (more than 103 degrees); and
- red, hot, and dry skin.

Heat Exhaustion

Heat exhaustion is a milder form of heat-related illness than heat stroke and is common among athletes. Signs include:

- goose bumps;
- heavy or light sweating;
- paleness;
- muscle cramps;
- tiredness, weakness;
- dizziness;
- headache;
- nausea or vomiting; and
- fainting.

Caffeine and Alcohol: Are They Dehydrating?

After much scientific debate, the Institute of Medicine in 2004 issued their hydration guidelines that approved caffeinated beverages and alcoholic beverages as options to count toward daily fluid needs. However, don't get too excited. While we believe both are fine to provide part of your daily fluid requirements, the side effects of too much caffeine (upset stomach, nervousness, irritability) or alcohol (drowsiness, inability to function and concentrate, loss of motor skills) won't serve you well as an athlete.

Many athletes we know can't race without their morning coffee, but few really go overboard with caffeinated beverages. And we have yet to find a professional athlete who has been successful using alcohol to stay hydrated or to rehydrate.

Buy a Better Sports Drink

Optimal carbohydrate concentration of sports drinks is 4 to 8 percent, or ten to eighteen grams of carbohydrate per eight-ounce serving. The one that works best for you may be the one that tastes best to you, so you actually will drink more of it. Also, recognize that your taste preferences will change depending on conditions, so what works for you in the cooler weather may not work as well in the heat of the summer. In ultraendurance events it's good to have several different flavors, as many athletes suffer from "flavor fatigue" and can become dehydrated as a result.

> To calculate the carbohydrate concentration of your favorite beverage, divide the number of grams of carbohydrate in an eight-ounce serving by 240 and then multiply by 100.

Sports drinks with lots of extra ingredients are not necessary and have not been proven to enhance endurance. If a product contains protein, taurine, choline, ribose, ginseng, glucosamine, or creatine, you probably are paying more for an ingredient(s) that has not been sufficiently proven to enhance performance in a sports drink. In addition, these added ingredients may slow the digestion and absorption of carbohydrates and fluids, so it's best to stick with products that deliver what you need most—fluid, carbohydrates, and sodium.

When reading the ingredients list, make sure that glucose, maltodextrin, sucrose, or dextrose are listed before fructose, indicating that they are in much higher concentration in the beverage. It's also worth reading manufacturers' Web sites to get more information on the proportion or ratio of the types of sugars in their products.

Product	CHO 8 ounces	CHO Concentration 8 ounces	Sodium 8 ounces	Calories 8 ounces	Sugar Source
PowerBar Endurance	17 g	7	190 mg	70	Maltodextrin, fructose, and dextrose blend

Product	CHO 8 ounces	CHO Concentration 8 ounces	Sodium 8 ounces	Calories 8 ounces	Sugar Source
Gatorade Endurance Formula	14 g	6	200 mg	50	Sucrose, glucose, and fructose blend
Gatorade Thirst Quencher	14 g	6	110 mg	50	Sucrose, glucose, and fructose blend
Accelerade	15 g	6	120 mg	80	Contains protein, sucrose, fructose, and maltodextrin
Cytomax Performance Drink	10 g	5	40 mg	50	Maltodextrin, fructose, dextrose
PowerAde	15 g	6	53 mg	57	Sucrose maltodextrin
Gu20	13 g	5	120 mg	50	Maltodextrin, fructose
Clif Shot Electrolyte	19 g	8	200 mg	80	Brown rice syrup and cane juice

Cramps 101

The sudden, intense pain that can virtually cripple you in seconds is often attributed to dehydration, sodium, or electrolyte imbalances, but there is substantial evidence to suggest that unless an athlete has severe dehydration or sodium losses, then muscle overload, muscle fatigue, or a breakdown in communication between muscles and nerves is more likely the cramp culprit. Cramps related to severe dehydration and low sodium tends to be more severe and involve many muscle groups rather than only the exercising muscle.

To avoid cramps, follow standard exercise protocols and don't exceed a 10 percent jump in duration or intensity at any given time. Also, sudden changes in speed or terrain in the later stages of exercise often precipitate a cramp, so ease into a faster pace, and when terrain changes (e.g., level to hills), when you feel the first signs of cramps, generally muscle twinges or twitches precipitate full-blown cramps. Drinking 8 to 16 ounces of a sports drink or water with 180 mg sodium (about 1 salt tablet) or a few pinches of table salt has been suggested to help in some cases.

Carbohydrates during Exercise

Now that you understand your hydration needs, the next order of business is your carbohydrate requirements. Most of us have about two thousand calories' worth of stored carbohydrates among what's stored in our liver, muscles, and blood to use during exercise. That will last about sixty to ninety minutes, depending on how big you are and the intensity of the exercise. An hour of high-intensity exercise has been shown to burn through 55 percent of liver glycogen, and in two hours, that glycogen is kaput. This is why athletes can get by with only water when exercising less than an hour; but go longer, and they'll need additional carbohydrates to keep the pace and intensity levels high.

Hundreds of studies have shown that carbohydrates consumed during exercise delay fatigue in endurance athletes, but carbohydrates during exercise also are important for athletes in high-intensity stop-and-go sports such as soccer, ice hockey, tennis, basketball, baseball, and football, as well as in precision sports. Carbohydrate consumption during all sports can help ward off fatigue within muscles but also the mental fatigue that can be associated with sports requiring lots of concentration. Remember, the brain is the hungriest of all organs for glucose. In fact, the brain is twenty to thirty times more metabolically active than muscles, and unlike other tissues, the brain can utilize only glucose for fuel.

Studies also have found that there is an upper limit to how much carbohydrate will be burned as fuel, even when more carbs are ingested. The rate of stomach emptying and intestinal absorption of carbohydrates appears to have limits as to how much carbohydrate can be absorbed per minute. It appears that 1 gram per minute is the upper limit, but newer studies suggest that this may be increased substantially with training and by the delivery and type of carbohydrate consumed.

As a general rule, sports nutritionists and the American College of Sports Medicine recommend the following:

30 to 60 grams of carbohydrates per hour

120 to 240 carbohydrate calories per hour

This recommendation, as you can see, is fairly general and equals a 120-calorie difference per hour. For athletes exercising at high intensity and burning through carbs at a rate of 4 grams per minute or 240 grams an hour, you can see it doesn't take too long to burn through all the available carbs the body has stored and then some. When exercising for more than an hour, it's essential to take in additional carbohydrates to maintain the speed or power or intensity.

There are also newer data questioning if 60 grams of carbohydrates per hour is really the upper limit that athletes can burn. Despite the concern that more carbs could delay stomach emptying and increase GI discomfort, the glucose/fructose blend appears to be faring quite well—similar to water. As a general rule, athletes exercising at lower intensities can tolerate higher amounts of carbohydrates because there is more blood flow to the GI tract and less in the muscles compared to individuals working out at higher intensities.

The best way to determine what works best is to start with 30 to 60 grams of CHO per hour and increase or decrease intake according to how you feel and how well you perform. If you are a larger athlete, you require more energy and should strive for the higher carbohydrate goals compared to a lighter athlete. Use the table on page 118 as a general guideline to determine how much carbohydrate to strive for during exercise. We have broken it into categories based on body weight, as that is one way to better tailor carbohydrate guidelines. However, we have seen female Ironman competitors who weigh a feathery 110 pounds (soaking wet) who can tolerate more than 90 grams of carbs per hour on the bike portion of the triathlon. That said, use this as a starting point and tweak your carbohydrate intake upward or downward based on how you feel and perform during exercise.

We suggest keeping a workout log when dialing in your carbohydrate needs. In it, track the workout and everything you ate and drank during the workout. Record your times, splits, how you felt on a scale of 1 to 10, and any GI issues. Repeat that same workout once a month, change the carbohydrate intake, and record the same measures as before. Many elite-level athletes we work with do this to dial in their nutrition before key events. They also tell us that their body adapts to higher carbohydrate intake as the season progresses and they practice consuming more in training.

To get those carbs in you, it's best to stick with the most digestible carb-rich options available. Your sports nutrition arsenal can include sport bars, sport drinks, gels, and real food. Use the chart on page 119 for the best ways to use different sports nutrition products.

Duration of Exercise/Event	Carbohydrate Requirements
Under 1 hour	Water or sports drinks only; additional carbohydrates unnecessary
1 to 2 hours	Carbs at 30 to 60 grams per hour
	<130 pounds, 30 grams
	>150 pounds, 60 grams
2+ hours	Carbs at 45 to 90 grams per hour
	<130 lbs, 45 grams
	>150 lbs, 90 grams
4+ hour	Carbs at 45 to 100* grams per hour

*Research reveals that by consuming multiple sources of carbohydrates, with primary sources being glucose, maltodextrin, and other simple sugars, and fructose as the secondary carbohydrate source in a 2:1 ratio, you can take in more grams of carbohydrate and your body is able to use more carbohydrate per hour. It is suggested that the body uses dual transport mechanisms to absorb fructose compared to other simple sugars and therefore can burn substantially more than 60 grams of carbohydrates per hour. Some studies have found that a glucose-fructose combination can boost carb combustion by 20 percent or more compared to a glucose-only feeding.

Energy Bars

Since the inception of the PowerBar Performance Bar in the 1984, there are now hundreds of energy bars available, many of which claim to have miraculous ingredients to enhance performance. There are "women-only," high-protein, meal-replacement bars and endurance-focused bars or those for power athletes, so it's hard to determine what you really need.

Look for a bar that is high in carbohydrates relative to the protein and fat content. Since protein and fat slow digestion, only individuals exercising in longer-duration, lower-intensity events tend to be able to eat protein- or fat-rich bars while exercising. Some bars, such as PowerBar Performance Bars, provide 60 percent or more of their calories from carbohydrates. Other bars are too high in protein or fat.

Since the goal of an energy bar should be to help you meet your carbohydrate goals per hour, add the carbs from the bar you choose to the carbs consumed with a sports drink to calculate your total carbohydrate consumption per hour. Generally, the higher the intensity of exercise, the more you will rely on fluid sources of carbohydrates. Individuals who rely on bars for most of their carbohydrates tend to be active people who may be exercising at a lower intensity, or doing endurance events where they need more variety in their fueling options. To enhance gastric emptying of the bar and to minimize GI distress, be sure to drink plenty of water with the bar to try to get the carbohydrate concentration lower for maximum rate of uptake.

Buying a Better Energy Bar

- Choose bars that provide the majority of their calories from carbohydrates—more than 70 percent of calories—with smaller amounts of protein and fat, both of which are slower to digest.
- Bars with more grams of fiber may cause GI problems during exercise, so look for those with modest amounts of fiber.

Product (size)	Calories	Carbs (g)	Protein (g)	Fat (g)	Fiber (g)	Notes
PowerBar Performance Vanilla Crisp (65 g)	240	45	8	3.5	1	200 mg sodium, organic, evaporated cane juice syrup, maltodextrin and fructose, fortified
PowerBar Harvest Peanut Butter Chocolate Chip (65 g)	240	42	10	4.5	5	140 mg sodium, brown rice syrup, cane juice syrup, fortified
Clif Bar Energy Bar Chocolate Chip Peanut Crunch (68 g)	250	43	11	6	5	125 mg sodium, organic brown rice syrup, cane juice, fortified
Balance Bar Peanut Butter (50 g)	200	22	14	6	1	230 mg sodium, fortified, high-fructose corn syrup
Snickers Marathon Energy Bar Chewy Chocolate Peanut (55 g)	210	25	14	8	4	Corn syrup, sugar, fortified
LaraBar Cashew Cookie (48 g)	200	25	6	12	4	Dates are sugar source
Odwalla Bar! Chocolate Chip Peanut Butter (62 g)	250	38	8	7	4	80 mg sodium, brown rice syrup, fortified, cane juice
Tiger's Milk King-Size Peanut Butter (55 g)	230	28	9	10	1	125 mg sodium, high-fructose corn syrup, fortified
Balance Bar Gold Caramel Nut Blast	210	24	13	7	0	150 mg sodium

- Look for products that provide multiple carbohydrate sources but more glucose or maltodextrin or dextrose than fructose. Research suggests that a 2:1 ratio of glucose to fructose may enhance endurance performance.

- Please your taste buds. If you don't like the bar, you won't eat it.

- Is it edible in your conditions? Some bars melt in the heat, and others are too hard to bite into during the cold; make sure your bar works in the environment in which you train and compete.

> *Energy to Burn Nutritionism:* To calculate the percentage of calories from carbs in a bar, multiply the grams of carbohydrates by 4 and divide by calories in the bar.

Energy Gels

For times when carrying sports drinks is out of the question, a quick and easy way to get a dose of carbs is with energy gels. As a cross between a sports bar and a sports drink, look for gels that provide about twenty-five grams of carbohydrates (a hundred calories) as well as sodium. To dilute them to the optimal 4 to 8 percent carbohydrate concentration, you need to drink most gels with ten to twelve ounces of water. There is evidence to suggest that gels with a 2:1 ratio of glucose to fructose may enhance energy delivery, allowing you to consume more carbs per hour without GI discomfort.

Caffeine is also in some flavors of energy gels. For example, some flavors of PowerBar Gel contain fifty milligrams of caffeine, or about half as much caffeine as a cup of coffee. There is evidence to suggest that caffeine acts as an ergogenic aid and helps to delay fatigue. Like sports bars and drinks, there's no need for your gel to have unnecessary ingredients that have not been proven to enhance performance.

Gel (size)	Calories	Carbs (g)	Protein (g)	Sodium (mg)	Carb Source	Other
PowerBar Gel (41g)	110–120	27–28	—	200	Maltodextrin, fructose	Specific flavors contain 25 or 50 mg of caffeine
GU Energy Gel (32 g)	100	25	—	40–55	Maltodextrin, fructose	Specific flavors contain caffeine fortified with vitamins C and E

Gel (size)	Calories	Carbs (g)	Protein (g)	Sodium (mg)	Carb Source	Other
GU Roctane (32 g)	100	25	—	65	Maltodextrin, fructose	Includes BCAA, 35 mg of caffeine
Clif Shot Gel	100	25	—	40	Brown rice syrup	Specific flavors contain caffeine
Accel Gel (41 g)	100	20	5	100	Sucrose, fructose	Some have caffeine fortified with vitamins C and E
E* Gel (55 g)	150	37		230	Maltodextrin, fructose	No caffeine, fortified with vitamins C, E, and B
Hammer Gel (36 g)	90	23	—	25–45	Maltodextrin, fruit concentrates	Amino acids

Multiday Events: Fuel Up or Fry

The longer the event, the more important nutrition becomes. In fact, among professional cyclists in the Tour de France, poor nutrition and dehydration are two of the leading causes for dropping out of the race.

We had the chance to work with several professional cyclists about their nutrition for stage races. If you can imagine, these athletes need to consume up to 50 percent of their total daily calories while riding a bike at twenty-five to thirty miles per hour in a tight, testosterone-packed peloton. And that's no easy feat, considering that these athletes can burn about seven thousand calories a day. Here's a breakdown of the caloric requirements for the Tour of California stages in 2007 and what it would equal in calories.

2007 Amgen Tour of California Stage-by-Stage Energy Costs

Energy cost of stage one: Sausalito to Santa Rosa (100 miles) = 3,400 calories

Caloric equivalent: seven and a half PowerBar Performance Bars and ten 20-ounce bottles of PowerBar Endurance or other fluid electrolyte beverage

Energy cost of stage two: Santa Rosa to Sacramento (116 miles) = 4,000 calories

Caloric equivalent: Two 12-inch Domino's pepperoni and cheese pizzas

Energy cost of stage three: Stockton to San Jose (95 miles) = 3,200 calories

Caloric Equivalent: seven and a half 20-ounce bottles of PowerBar Endurance and fifteen PowerBar Gels

Energy cost of stage four: Seaside to San Luis Obispo (134 miles) = 4,600 calories

Caloric equivalent: eight Burger King Double Cheeseburgers and a side of large fries

Energy cost of stage five: Solvang Time Trial (15 miles) = 500 calories

Caloric equivalent: two and a half 20-ounce bottles of PowerBar Endurance

Energy cost of stage six: Santa Barbara to Santa Clarita (105 miles) = 3,500 calories

Caloric equivalent: Ten 20-ounce water bottles with PowerBar Endurance Sport Drink and sixteen PowerBar Gels

Energy cost of stage seven: Long Beach Circuit Race (77 miles) = 2,800 calories

Caloric equivalent: twenty-eight large bananas

Minimizing GI Distress: Gut-Friendly Tips for Endurance Athletes

Almost every endurance and ultraendurance athlete we know has complained about GI distress. Whether you are running a marathon or ultra, a triathlon or adventure race, GI problems are among the most common reasons why endurance athletes drop out of races or have subpar performances. Having to make repeat Porta Potty stops can turn any type of challenging endurance event into a death march.

One study found that among Ironman competitors, 93 percent experienced some type of GI symptom during the race (including reflux, gas, bloating, nausea, vomiting). Among those with GI symptoms, 45 percent said that their symptoms were severe, and 7 percent were forced to abandon the race due to their symptoms.

The good news is that most GI problems are avoidable, and proper nutrition training can help ensure that you can race without needing a plumber to clean out your pipes all day. An easy way to minimize the likelihood of having a problem is to practice your race day nutrition strategies in training, and don't do anything new prior to and during your race. If you suffer from GI problems in training, keep a log of the symptoms and what you ate and drank during training. Your log can help you identify the culprit or culprits.

Below are the key culprits causing GI distress and what you can do to best avoid succumbing to your stomach.

Follow a Hydration Schedule

The stomach and the GI tract work best when they have adequate fluids in them, and being dehydrated will slow stomach emptying, making you feel bloated and giving you the "stomach slosh" effect and other GI symptoms. The key is to avoid becoming dehydrated during exercise by calculating your personal hydration zone and keeping within it.

Keep Concentrated Carbs in Check

When taking in your carbohydrate calories during the race, make sure to keep them at their optimal concentration. To do that, mix your sports drinks according to labels, and whenever you take a bar or a gel, be sure to drink the recommended fluid intake with it. If you choose to eat foods, be sure to take eight ounces of water or sports drink with solids to keep the carbohydrate concentration in check.

Sodium Solutions

By using higher-sodium sports drinks and gels, you should be able to keep your sodium levels adequate during endurance and ultraendurace training and racing. Most athletes strive for 500 mg to 1,000 mg (1 g) sodium per hour. You can easily accomplish this with, for example, two PowerBar Gels (200 mg of sodium per packet) and 16 ounces of PowerBar Endurance sport drink (380 mg of sodium) totaling 780 mg of sodium as well as 96 g of carbohydrates.

Too much sodium, however, or too much of any of the electrolytes can lead to bloating, nausea, and vomiting, so be sure to practice with your sodium intake during exercise to drill down to your optimal sodium intake per hour of exercise.

OTC Meds for Peace of Mind

Diarrhea is the most common concern on the run portion of an event, and Imodium can offer a great solution and serve as peace of mind. If you are prone to diarrhea while running, taking two antidiarrheal medicine (e.g., Imodium) an hour or so before the start of your event. Many athletes carry OTC antidiarrheal meds with them on course as well. Also, putting the OTC products in your special-needs bag and on your bike will provide added peace of mind.

RACE-DAY GI PROBLEMS AND SOLUTIONS

Problem	Solution
Race day stress, anxiety	Choose liquid meal rather than solids on race morning; use relaxation techniques.
Too many calories before and during	Stick with tried-and-true prerace and race-day fueling strategies. Devise a plan, practice it in training, and execute it on race day.
Excess caffeine	Practice your race-day caffeine intake at "B" races or in training to determine your threshold.
High fiber	Switch to a low-fiber diet two to three days prior to the race; have white breads, reduce fruit and vegetables, and have more juices and processed low-fiber foods.
Too-high intensity	Too-high intensity impedes the GI tract from functioning, so race at the right intensity; slow down if you are going hard and having GI problems.
Aspirin and NSAIDs	Eliminate two to three days prior to the race; take during the race only if 100 percent necessary.

To avoid GI problems, stick to the sports nutrition golden rule: never try anything new on race day. The second rule is to have a hydration and carbohydrate intake strategy in place that has worked in training, and stick to it on race day.

To avoid race day stomach troubles be sure that you start your race with adequate carbohydrate stores. Being fully hydrated is key, then maintaining good fluid status during the race. The stomach and the GI tract work best when there is some fluid and food in them at all times. If you're planning on using electrolyte supplements during the race, make sure you

---

**HINTS FROM ELITE-LEVEL ATHLETES WHO DOUBLE
AS SPORTS DIETITIANS**

Athlete: Kelly White, M.S., R.D., C.S.S.D., registered dietitian and Hawaii Ironman World Championship 2007 finisher

Event: Ironman Distance

Per Hour on the Bike	*Per Hour on the Run*
20 oz Endurance Beverage on course	20 oz water
	6 oz cola
½ PowerBar Performance Bar	6 oz Endurance Beverage
12 oz water	1 PowerBar Gel
	Handful of pretzels
Fluid ounces: 32	
Carbohydrates: 74 grams	Fluid ounces: 32
	Carbohydrates: 70 grams

---

have practiced with them beforehand, as too much sodium or potassium can cause bloating and diarrhea.

If your stomach acts up en route, don't despair. Slow your pace—pushing at too high of an intensity than you can handle can often lead to stomach problems as well. Assess your hydration and carbohydrate status and focus on addressing which may be contributing to the problem. More often it is due to inadequate hydration and carbohydrate intake, but sometimes it can be from overdoing calories during the race.

8

Optimal Recovery: Replenish, Repair, and Rehydrate

For me, the difference between being a hard-working age grouper and an Ironman world champion was proper recovery.

—*Peter Reid, three-time Ironman world champion*

AFTER AN EVENT . . .

Step one: Throw your arms up, holler "whoo-hoo!," look for friends and family, put the medal around your neck.

Step two: Grab a water bottle.

Step three: Look for food.

It is this last step that we often overlook after crossing the finish line. However satisfying the hugs and the kisses are, the fluid and food will arguably provide the most benefit. Not only will a smart recovery strategy make you feel better, it also will help you get over the physical stress of the day, replenish lost stores, repair muscle, rehydrate, and get you ready for your next adventure. After you exhaust yourself, or even after a moderate exercise bout, your body is ready to rebuild and rehydrate. It's essential that you give it the tools it needs to do so.

Energy to Burn Nutritionism: It can take twenty-four hours to replenish glycogen stores after depletion by exercise.

Your Body Is Ready to Rebuild

As we said, it's so important to recover properly after an exercise session. Your body agrees, and to show it, it readies itself to do so. After a workout, the body is primed for rebuilding. Some of the physiological changes that take place are:

- Glucose transporters are ready to carry glucose to the muscles for storage.
- There is an increase in enzymes that promote storage.
- Hormones that stimulate storage are at higher levels.

Glycogen is the primary fuel that drives your muscles during endurance exercise. After a day of training, your muscle and liver glycogen stores are low. After your stores are depleted, it can take a while to recover. To speed glycogen reloading you need to consume carbs as soon as possible after exercise. Storage rates are fastest in the first hour after exercise. Failing to consume carbs after exercise leads to very low rates of glycogen restoration until feeding does occur. In the first one to two hours, the stores can recover by about 7 to 8 percent; then they slow to 5 percent per hour thereafter.

Protein for Recovery

After a workout, not only do you need to consider the glycogen you used, but also the muscles you would like to repair, and in the case of resistance training, grow. Researchers have looked at glycogen replenishment and the role that protein plays, with mixed results. If you are consuming enough carbs after exercise, protein may not improve glycogen replenishment. But you definitely need protein in recovery to repair those muscles.

The second aim is to recover from the stress on the muscles. Researchers have identified benefits from ten grams of protein with eight grams of carbohydrates in a beverage when the measure of interest was whole-body protein-building. Although more research is warranted, it is safe to say that protein after exercise is a good idea.

Last, protein may be a valuable addition to your snack or meal following a resistance training session. Even a small amount of amino acids then appears to stimulate protein-building and therefore benefits muscle repair and growth. The good news is that you don't have to consume massive amounts of protein to achieve this benefit; even a small amount (e.g., six grams of protein) can be helpful for the first several hours following a session.

For strength and resistance, new research shows that for optimal muscle growth after a workout, a slightly higher protein intake range is beneficial. To optimize muscle growth, consume between 0.05 and 0.18 grams per pound of body weight (0.1 to 0.4 grams per kg) within four hours of training.

Fat for Recovery?

While carbs and protein are certainly dietary priorities for athletes, don't forgo healthy fats during recovery. Your muscles contain lipid droplets or small deposits of fat called intramyocellular lipids or IMCL. Scientists theorize that these muscle lipids may be important sources of muscle fuel early in exercise, which may help spare muscle glycogen stores for later. These muscle lipids get depleted during endurance exercise, and many endurance athletes eat very-low-fat diets in their quest to consume enough carbs, causing them to fall short of meeting their daily needs for lipid reloading during recovery.

- Healthy fat sources in the diet to aid in recovery include olive oil, canola oil, and fats from nuts and avocados.
- A PowerBar Recovery Bar after exercise is a convenient option that provides thirty grams of carbohydrates to help replenish glycogen stores, twelve grams of protein to help support muscle tissue repair and building, and nine to ten grams of a lipid blend to help with muscle lipid reloading.

Time Your Recovery

We think it's most helpful to get to the nuts and bolts of recovery and give you clear recommendations for what to eat and when. We want to break it down by time so you can plan ahead and focus on your performance, rather than your confusion about what to eat after an important workout.

Zero to Thirty Minutes Postexercise

What: Carbohydrates

Why: Replenish glycogen stores

How much: 0.5 multiplied by your weight in pounds = grams of carbs
   Example: If you weigh 150 pounds, you need 75 grams of carbohydrates ($150 \times 0.5 = 75$).

What: Proteins

Why: The amino acids in the proteins you eat are used to make new proteins for muscle tissue repair and the building of new muscle as part of adapting to the physiologic demands of exercise.

How much: Consume ten to twenty grams of protein as soon as possible after training for muscle tissue repair and building.

SAMPLE POSTEXERCISE SNACK OPTIONS

Food Items and Meal Ideas	Kcals	Carb (g)	Protein (g)	Fat (g)
3 mini cinnamon-raisin bagels spread with 1 tbsp low-fat cream cheese 1 cup fresh blueberries 8 oz herbal tea	365	73	10.6	5
1 cup wheat (bran) flakes cereal sprinkled with ¼ cup ground almonds 1 cup skim milk 1 cup strawberry halves	392	59	18.4	13.6
1 whole grain English muffin, toasted 1 tbsp vegetable spread 1 cup low-fat, fruit-on-the-bottom yogurt 1 small, fresh orange	527	92	18	10

Breakfast sandwich
  2 slices whole-wheat bread, toasted
  2 tsp vegetable spread
  1 poached egg
½ cup fresh baby spinach
1 cup grapefruit sections
2 medium tomato slices
	520	74	25	15

¾ cup low-fat cottage cheese mixed with ¾ cup each fresh strawberries and blueberries 1 oz hard pretzels	325	50	25	4
1 PowerBar Harvest Bar, apple cinnamon flavor 8 oz spiced herbal tea	240	42	10	4
1 oat bran bagel spread with ⅓ cup marinara sauce and 1 oz low-fat mozzarella cheese	262	37	15.3	6

Shake
  2 tbsp whey protein powder, any flavor
  1 medium banana
  2 tbsp fat-free chocolate syrup
	420	77	19	4

Food Items and Meal Ideas	Kcals	Carb (g)	Protein (g)	Fat (g)
8 oz skim milk ½ cup crushed ice				
Open-face sandwich 1 slice whole grain bread topped with 1 tbsp hummus and 1 oz each of deli roast beef, chicken, and lean ham	211	19	23	5
1 PowerBar Triple Threat Bar, S'mores flavor 1 medium banana	344	57	11	8
8 oz light yogurt mixed with 2 tbsp flax seeds, 1 sliced kiwi fruit, and 1 cup chopped apple	354	64	8	9

Up to Two Hours Postexercise

What: Carbohydrates

How much: 0.5 × your weight in pounds = grams of carbs (See the example above.)

Recovery Meals to Try

Simple sandwich

1 whole-wheat bagel
2 tsp Dijon mustard
1 tbsp mayonnaise
3 oz lean turkey

2 lettuce leaves
2 slices of tomato
5 dill pickle slices

1 cup mandarin oranges, canned in juice

1 fruit leather bar

Nutrition Facts	Total kilocalories: 618 Grams of carbohydrate: 92.6	Grams of protein: 31.6 Grams of fat: 15.5

Macaroni and cheese

1½ cups cooked, whole-wheat
  macaroni
½ cup shredded, low-fat cheddar
  cheese

½ cup 1% milk
1½ cups broccoli, chopped, cooked

1 cup diced pineapple

Nutrition Facts	Total kilocalories: 654 Grams of carbohydrate: 97	Grams of protein: 38.5 Grams of fat: 17.5

Nutty oatmeal

1 cup oatmeal made from ⅓ cup
dry oats and ¾ cup skim milk

1 tbsp natural peanut butter (mixed
into oatmeal)

1 medium banana
10 oz skim milk

| *Nutrition* | Total kilocalories: 464 | Grams of protein: 25 |
| *Facts* | Grams of carbohydrate: 72 | Grams of fat: 10.8 |

Toast with egg whites

2 slices 100 percent whole-wheat
toast
1 tbsp reduced-fat spread

1 tbsp 100 percent fruit preserves
2 egg whites cooked in 1 tbsp
reduced-fat spread

1 cup cantaloupe, cubed
6 oz nonfat, light yogurt

| *Nutrition* | Total kilocalories: 448 | Grams of protein: 19.6 |
| *Facts* | Grams of carbohydrate: 70.5 | Grams of fat: 11.3 |

Pita packed with tuna salad

1 whole-wheat pita
Tuna salad:
 ½ cup tuna, canned in water,
 drained
 3 tbsp reduced-fat mayonnaise
 2 tsp Dijon mustard

2 small dill pickles, chopped
3 large green olives, chopped
¼ cup chopped green bell pepper
2 lettuce leaves
2 slices of tomato

12 fl oz fresh orange juice

| *Nutrition* | Total kilocalories: 640 | Grams of protein: 30 |
| *Facts* | Grams of carbohydrate: 89 | Grams of fat: 21 |

Almond butter pancakes with blueberries

2 4-inch pancakes, from frozen batter
2 tbsp natural almond butter

2 tbsp pancake syrup
½ cup fresh blueberries

8 oz skim milk

| *Nutrition* | Total kilocalories: 540 | Grams of protein: 20 |
| *Facts* | Grams of carbohydrate: 79 | Grams of fats 18 |

Within Twenty-four Hours

If you have twenty-four hours or more to recover between training sessions, total carbohydrate intake, rather than timing of intake, is the more important issue for replenishing glycogen stores.

- Light training: About 3 grams of carbs per pound of body weight are needed over the next twenty-four hours. For example, if you weigh 150 pounds (150 × 3 = 450), consume 450 grams of carbs over the next twenty-four hours.
- Moderate-to-heavy endurance training: About 4 grams of carbs per pound of body weight are needed daily.
- Extreme training (equal to or greater than four hours per day): About 5 grams of carbs per pound of body weight are needed daily.
- Consume a mix of quick- and slower-to-digest carbohydrate sources, including fruits, vegetables, breads, cereals, pasta, rice, potatoes, and beans. Recovery bars and beverages are also fine to consume.

Don't Forget to Rehydrate

If you ran in the Boston Marathon in 2008, you may not have been surprised to find a handout titled "The Right Way to Hydrate for a Marathon" in your welcome packet. Following the abruptly canceled, heat-affected 2007 Chicago Marathon, many endurance races began to supply entrants with information on the art of hydration. Developed by the American Medical Athletic Association, the brochure offered pertinent information on the art of prerace and event-day hydration. What was lacking was extensive information on the art of rehydration.

Rehydration: What's the Big Deal?

It seems that information abounds concerning how much, and what, to drink before and during an event. What is often overlooked is the need to rehydrate. We know what it's like: you finish the workout of your life and all you want to do is hit the shower and then the couch. It's hard enough taking in those carbs and protein necessary to recovery, let alone fluids. So why is rehydration a big deal? It's a big deal because most athletes will replace only 30 to 70 percent of the total fluid they lose during exercise, and most active individuals will lose one to four liters of fluid per hour during exercise, depending on event intensity, weather conditions, and various physiological parameters. Based on the above stats, it is likely that once you finish a strenuous workout or a long-distance event, you are somewhat, if not very, dehydrated. So just as important as preevent fueling and during-event hydration is postevent rehydration.

Hydration following exercise of any sort is of extreme importance. Granted, if you just went for a walk around the block in fifty-degree temperatures, you can get away with skipping an ounce or two of water. But turn that neighborhood block into fifteen miles, the fifty degrees into eighty degrees, skip rehydration, and you're doomed because dehydration equals impaired performance and health.

Sodium also is important and relates to fluid needs, as it's lost in sweat and usually consumed in sports beverages. Sodium not only maintains plasma osmolality and wards off hyponatremia, but also the additional sodium in foods triggers the thirst response, prompting you to drink more fluids.

We've convinced you it's important; now here's how to rehydrate.

How to Rehydrate

Whether your next big event is a marathon or a leisurely bike ride, it takes some planning ahead to make sure you're hydrated and ready to go. You don't want to face your next workout still in fluid debt (aka dehydrated) from your previous one. If you have plenty of time between events, you can rehydrate more leisurely. But should your next event or workout be within the next twelve hours, or if you've lost excessive fluid (more than 2 percent of your body weight), you need a strategy for rapid rehydration:

- Drink about twenty-three ounces of fluid per pound of weight lost during exercise.
- Drink gradually between the end of your first workout and one to two hours before the start of your next workout.
- Fluids containing sodium, an electrolyte that is vital to recovery, will expedite recovery by not only retaining fluids but also by stimulating the thirst mechanism.
- Fluids that contain other necessary electrolytes—chloride and potassium—also can be beneficial.
- Sports drinks are your friend; these drinks contain not only desirable electrolytes, they also multitask. With added carbs, sports drinks help you to refuel while helping you to rehydrate.
- Drinks with added herbs, supplements, and vitamins are not needed.

You don't lose vitamins when you sweat. And you certainly don't lose ginkgo biloba, chromium, or passion fruit extract.

Here's an example of one rehydration strategy we created for a triathlete in training:

Training: Two-a-day

Day one: Ten-mile run, seventy-five-degree temperature

Day two: Thirty-mile bike ride, eighty-degree temperature

Strategy: Hydration starts before you head out the door for a run.

During the run, aim for consumption of eighteen to thirty-two ounces of water or sports drink per hour. Since a ten-mile run may take you longer than an hour, start drinking a sports drink before you reach the one-hour mark. Pay close attention to fluid intake toward the end of your run; you are essentially planning ahead for your next event.

Strategy: Hydration continues when you take off the running shoes.

After completing the run, consume twenty-three ounces of fluid for each pound of weight lost during the run. Aim for a fluid containing both calories from carbs and needed electrolytes.

Strategy: Begin the bike ride fully hydrated.

Most athletes find that this can be done by consuming two to three milliliters per pound at least four hours before the event. (Remember, there are thirty milliliters in one ounce.) If two hours before the ride, your urine is fairly dark, continue to drink more fluids.

Strategy: Don't forget about final rehydration.

Now that your two-a-day is completed, don't forget about rehydrating. Sure, you may not be heading out for another workout soon, but you still need to recover. If you're taking some time to rest and your next workout isn't for a day or so, see the following information on relaxed rehydration.

Relaxed Rehydration

If you're on the more leisurely path to recovery—that is, if you have twenty-four hours or more to rehydrate—normal consumption of beverages, meals, and snacks will generally return you to a hydrated state within twenty-four hours. Most food items contain a large percentage of water, and this water, in turn, is used by the body for hydration needs. In addition to muscle recovery and glycogen reuptake, another benefit to consuming a meal or a snack following exercise is that solid foods often can pack a large sodium punch and, as stated above, sodium is crucial to recovery of fluid status.

Monitor Your Progress

Following any event or workout, the best way to monitor if you've done a proper job rehydrating is to monitor your body weight and urine color. Your preworkout weight should be met, you should be within your hydration zone (see chapter 7 on hydration), and the color of your urine should range from light yellow to clear.

Summary of Recommendations

If you plan to train again in fewer than twelve hours, or if you've lost excessive fluid (more than 2 percent of your body weight), you need a strategy for rapid rehydration:

- Drink about twenty-three ounces of fluid per pound of weight lost during exercise. Drink gradually between the end of your first workout and one to two hours before the start of your next workout.

If you have twenty-four hours or more to rehydrate:

- Normal consumption of beverages, meals, and snacks will generally rehydrate you within about twenty-four hours.
- Monitor your body weight and urine color.
- Consume sources of sodium while you rehydrate. This will help you retain ingested fluids and help stimulate your thirst. You can obtain sodium from recovery beverages and bars, sports drinks, energy bars and gels, salty snacks, and meals.

So take care with your rehydration: exhausted or not when you finish your workout, push back the shower, walk past the couch, and turn on the faucet. You'll thank yourself the next time you hit the track, the trails, the court, or the road.

9

Supplements: Help or Hype?

Dietary supplement is "a food product, added to the total diet, that contains at least one of the following ingredients: a vitamin, mineral, herb or botanical, amino acid, metabolite, constituent, extract, or combination of these ingredients."
—*Dietary Supplement Health and Education Act*

Functional foods are "foods or dietary components that may provide a health benefit beyond basic nutrition."
—*International Food Information Council*

It only takes a quick internet search to see that there are an overwhelming number of supplements advertised as ways to prevent disease, treat sore muscles, promote wellness, or give you more energy. Keeping up with the latest and greatest, as well as the supporting research, can be a challenge, as products often hit the store shelves before the scientists evaluate their effectiveness. Slack rules and regulations exist to protect the consumer, but you can easily purchase products you don't need, or worse, you can pop some pills disguised as dietary supplements that may have detrimental effects.

Most athletes we know and counsel take some type of supplement, but not because we suggest that they do. In fact, one study found that when you include fortified bars and other products as supplements, 99 percent of elite athletes reported using some type of dietary supplements, and there are thousands from which to choose. Athletes take their pills daily, often for the wrong reasons or with unreasonable expectations. For the athlete, the consequences of using supplements also include disqualification and

Energy to Burn Nutritionism: In 2004, Americans spent $20.3 billion on dietary supplements. *(Nutrition Business Journal, 2005)*

penalties, since many substances are banned from competition. Surprisingly, some over-the-counter dietary supplements contain substances that have been banned from sports; therefore there is no guarantee that an over-the-counter supplement is a safe choice. For you elite athletes, talk to your coaches frequently about any supplements you take, and read the fine print on all your antidoping documents from your governing association (e.g., the International Olympic Committee or the National Collegiate Athletic Association). There isn't a performance-enhancing substance that will help you if you have been kicked off your team for breaking the rules.

Who's Making the Rules for Dietary Supplements?

As mentioned, there are rules that regulate dietary supplements—sort of. The Dietary Supplement Health Education Act (DSHEA) of 1994 created a definition for a dietary supplement and charged the Food and Drug Administration (FDA) with monitoring the safety of a supplement . . . *after* it reaches the market. The FDA is *not* responsible for analyzing the contents of a supplement or making sure that the supplement you purchase works. The way the act is designed, the manufacturer is responsible for ensuring that the supplement's label is truthful and not misleading. Manufacturers are also expected to follow the Good Manufacturing Practices (GMP), which ensures consistency in how the supplement is prepared, packed, and stored. According to the National Institutes of Health's Office of Dietary Supplements, there is no such thing as "standardization," as there is no accepted U.S. definition pertaining to dietary supplements. Therefore there is no assurance that each supplement has the same dose of active ingredients, nor any that it works.

Energy to Burn Nutritionism: According to the 2002 Health and Diet Survey, 73 percent of U.S. adults reported using a dietary supplement.

Here are the players in the dietary supplement regulatory world:

- Food and Drug Administration: Responsible for taking action against a supplement after it's on the market.
- Federal Trade Commission: Ensures that the advertising of dietary supplements in national or regional newspapers and magazines; in

radio and TV commercials, including infomercials; through direct mail to consumers; or on the Internet is not misleading and is truthful.

- Good Manufacturing Practices: Describes the conditions under which products must be prepared, packed, and stored.
- Office of Dietary Supplements: Office under the National Institutes of Health created in 1995 under the DSHEA to evaluate the science behind supplements, stimulate and support research, release research results, and educate the public.

You're on Your Own

With the FDA monitoring the safety of a supplement *after* it's in your kitchen cabinet (or even your gut) and the GMP giving us little confidence on all issues associated with quality, there are many reasons to be skeptical about supplements. If you still need to be convinced, here's a list of reasons why you need to do your own research before buying a supplement:

- The FDA does *not* ensure that your supplement is safe until *after* it hits the shelves.
- Unlike with drugs, manufacturers do *not* have to ensure that the supplement is safe (through research in humans) prior to selling.
- The FDA will take action against a supplement only after reports of adverse effects start rolling in.
- The buyer is expected to report adverse reactions to the FDA.
- The manufacturer does *not* have to make sure it works, nor is any agency or organization required to check to make sure that your supplement is effective.
- A "seal of approval" on the label means that the supplement has passed the manufacturer's quality testing. It does not say anything about its safety or effectiveness.
- Supplements are not intended to treat, diagnose, mitigate, prevent, or cure disease . . . yet they can have adverse effects.
- If you want to know if a particular brand is effective, contaminated, safe, or even contains what the label says it does, you are to call the manufacturer!

If It Quacks like a Duck . . .

When it comes to dietary supplements, as you can see, it's necessary to do your own research. Unfortunately, quack supplements abound. Quackery is so prevalent that the FDA has defined it! Quackery pertains not only to a person who is misrepresenting himself or herself (i.e., a pseudo-health care practitioner with faux credentials), but also to products that amount to nothing more than a waste of money. There are benefits to allowing consumers to take responsibility for their own purchases and health care—easier access to products, a greater understanding of personal needs, or more choices—but the sword is double-edged. With lax regulations designed to allow consumers to make their own decisions come a barrage of made-up stuff and fake claims. Save yourself some valuable time by scrolling through these telltale signs of quackery:

- Quick and easy: If the story leads with a health-related fix as being "quick and easy," it's likely not. Sure, some may feel that adding fruits and vegetables to their diet is quick and easy, but as a remedy for an ailment, quick and easy rarely fits the bill.

- Testimonials galore: Finding out what worked for others can be helpful, but we're all unique. Be skeptical and ask yourself, "Are these made-for-TV accounts?" or "Did she really lose ten pounds in two days?"

- The supplement is accompanied by a list of dietary and lifestyle modifications. Classic examples of this include weight-loss supplements that recommend a low-fat, reduced-calorie diet and daily exercise to achieve the benefits of the thirty-dollar-a-day supplement. Hmmm, could it be the former and not the latter? Save your money and see a dietitian and personal trainer.

- Right for everyone: Similar to the testimonial warning, not all supplements are right for everyone. You may have unique needs and pre-existing conditions as simple as intolerance to a substance that you may not be aware of.

- Used for millions of years: This is my personal favorite. Yes, it's impressive that it's been used as an ancient medical remedy and been around since the dinosaurs, but I'm pretty sure that even if you drive a hybrid, our lifestyle and environment are quite different from those in ancient times. I can't remember the last time I was hunting and gathering without a grocery cart, nor can I recall a day when I didn't inhale a pollutant or ingest a pesticide—never mind survive without caffeinated coffee or spend half my day staring at a computer screen. We can't hang our hat on that reasoning since we live and breathe in a much different environment today, and this may alter the impact an ancient remedy could have on our well-being.

- Position the health care and science community as villains. Among every group of board-certified health care professionals is a bad apple; that's not the issue. The issue is that using this scare tactic to sell a product is unethical and unfair. Capitalizing on fear and encouraging people to shirk off the recommendations of their physicians or debunk all science is unfounded and irresponsible. Science may not be perfect, it is a process and limited by funding and methodology, but its universal mission is *not* to spread misinformation and confusion. Nor are all physicians untrustworthy and villainous.

- Secret formulation: I'm not sure I want to ingest it if its contents are a secret. Is it a secret because it's a blend of pigs' feet and sedatives? It should cause a pause and then make you walk away—you need to know the ingredients before you pop it in your mouth.

- Pyramid scheme: Ask your doctor, your dietitian, your mom, and your accountant, should I invest a thousand dollars in this product and try to ruin my relationships with friends and family by pushing it on them at Thanksgiving and birthday parties? The answer is no. Overpriced opportunities to sell a supplement are rarely on the "up and up," as my mother would say.

Online Resources for Dietary Supplements

- Office of Dietary Supplements, NIH, HHS (http://ods.od.nih.gov/)
- Food and Nutrition Information Center (FNIC), USDA: Dietary Supplements and Herbal Information (www.nal.usda.gov/fnic/etext/000015.html)
- National Center for Complementary and Alternative Medicine (NCCAM), NIH, HHS (http://nccam.nih.gov/health/)
- Center for Food Safety and Applied Nutrition (CFSAN), FDA, HHS. Dietary Supplements: Consumer Education and General Information (www.cfsan.fda.gov/~dms/ds-info.html)
- International Bibliographic Information on Dietary Supplements (IBIDS) Database (http://grande.nal.usda.gov/ibids/index.php)
- Annual Bibliographies of Significant Advances in Dietary Supplement Research (http://ods.od.nih.gov/Research/Annual_Bibliographies.aspx)

- Dietary Supplement Fact Sheets (http://ods.od.nih.gov/Health_ Information/Information_About_Individual_Dietary_Supplements .aspx)
- NSF International, The Public Health and Safety Company (www.nsf.org)
- Informed Choice (www.informedchoice.org)
- World Anti-Doping Agency (WADA) (www.wada-ama.org)

Dietary Supplements for Performance: Ergogenic Aids

Among the dietary supplements reside a plethora of ergogenic aids. Ergogenic aids are intended to improve athletic performance. Ergogenic aids can be broken down into categories based on their purported effects, from biomechanical to psychological aids, but we'll focus on those that fall under the nutritional aids category. For these we have different types on the market that are intended to provide performance gains in a variety of ways:

- Antioxidants, vitamins, and minerals
- Strength and mass
- Endurance performance
- Fat loss
- Prevention of protein breakdown
- Androgenic effects
- Immune function

What's Out There?

There is a good chance that by the time you finish reading this section, another hot dietary supplement will hit the shelves. Some supplements have more research than others, while the evidence remains inconclusive for many. Let's look at what's out there and go through the proposed benefit (*They say* . . .), the evidence (*Science says* . . .), and we'll give you our thoughts whether we think it should be avoided or investigated (*We say* . . .). Please note that we will not prescribe any supplement to you—it's food first—and a prescription should be written by your doctor only. Our intention is to help you stay up to speed on what's on the shelves and where the research stands.

CHAT WITH AN EXPERT: CINCINNATI BENGALS' DIETITIAN MICHELE A. MACEDONIO, M.S., R.D., C.S.S.D., L.D.

1. What's your role with the Bengals?

   As the team dietitian for the Bengals, I deliver team presentations and meet one-on-one with players, helping them evaluate their eating behaviors and nutrient intake in relation to overall health, conditioning goals, and peak performance. From there we develop a nutrition strategy that will support goals for conditioning, training camp, and in-season performance. Nutrition education is the underpinning of all nutrition coaching so that players understand and buy into nutrition recommendations for modifications in food choices. Nutrition consultation may include making arrangements for dinner meals and may entail menu development, selecting personal chefs or other suitable options for dinners, providing recipes and cooking instructions for the players (and spouses/significant others) who prefer to cook their own meals, menu selection at restaurants, educational grocery shopping sessions, and the creation of written instructions and educational materials.

2. As a Board-certified specialist in sports dietetics working with professional athletes, are you frequently asked about dietary supplements to enhance performance?

   As a C.S.S.D., players feel confident asking me about supplements, knowing that I will research the product. I provide players with evidence-based information on supplements, addressing regulations, safety, adverse reactions, efficacy, cost/benefit ratio. The player can then make a determination as to taking a supplement or not. If a supplement is deemed safe and legal, I will provide information on known safe and efficacious doses.

3. What are the most common reasons why an athlete will ask about a supplement?

   Increasing muscle mass, promoting recovery (from intense training and from injury), "improved performance," "improved nutrition" are generally the reasons stated for inquiring about supplements.

4. What is your opinion on dietary supplements for athletes? Are there any that you recommend?

   My philosophy is "food first." I regard supplements as just that, supplements to the diet. If an athlete cannot or will not consume a diet that is adequate in energy and all essential nutrients, I will recommend an appropriate supplement to round out the diet. If an athlete has a particular need and it is not being met solely by diet, a supplement may fill that need. I look for wholesome products whose ingredients are considered safe and reliable. I regularly recommend particular food products as appropriate, some of which are considered functional foods.

Multivitamins

They say . . . A multivitamin (M/V) is an insurance plan to make sure you have the nutrients you need. An M/V will give you more energy if you're feeling run down and may improve performance.

Science says . . . Let's get straight to the point: there is no evidence that an M/V will improve athletic performance, only that antioxidants may help with damage caused by the stress of exercise. And even if you need a vitamin or mineral supplement, there is a tolerable upper intake level (UL) to the amount that can be safely consumed. More is

> *Energy to Burn Nutritionism:* An estimated 85 percent of supplement users take a multivitamin/multimineral supplement.

not necessarily better with vitamins and minerals; therefore it's important to review the label to ensure that you are near to the recommended dietary allowance (RDA) and not outrageously exceeding it. Over the years these recommendations have changed, so review the table on page 145 to see where we are now.

We say . . . So, as the Bengals' dietitian said, "food first," but some groups may benefit from an M/V. Vitamins and minerals are in a variety of foods, and depending on your current diet, an M/V may be helpful to ensure that you meet your needs. Here are groups that will benefit most from including an M/V:

- Those pregnant or lactating
- Those with diseases or disorders that increase needs
- Those using medications
- The elderly
- Vegans (no milk, no eggs)
- Those with restricted energy intake or those physically active but without adequate intake
- Those with food intolerances
- Those who make poor dietary choices

> "I take daily multivitamins (Centrum) and usually supplement it with some extra vitamin C."
> —Paul Fritzsche, professional triathlete and coach

COMPARISON OF 1989 RDA AND DRI VALUES FOR SELECTED NUTRIENTS

(Note: values in bold-faced type are previous or current RDA values. Values in plain type with an * indicate AI values.)

	1989 RDA Ages 19–50		New RDA or AI* Ages 19–50		UL[†] 19–70
	Women	Men	Women	Men	Men & Women
Vitamin A (µg/d)[1]	**800**	**1,000**	**700**	**900**	3,000
Vitamin C (mg/d)	**60**	**60**	**75**	**90**	2,000
Vitamin D (µg/d)	**5–10**[2]	**5–10**[2]	5*	5*	50
Vitamin E (mg/d)[3]	**8**	**10**	**15**	**15**	1,000[4]
Vitamin K (µg/d)	**60–65**[5]	**70–80**[5]	90*	120*	ND[6]
Thiamin (mg/d)	**1.1**	**1.5**	**1.1**	**1.2**	ND
Riboflavin (mg/d)	**1.3**	**1.7**	**1.1**	**1.3**	ND
Niacin (mg/d)[7]	**15**	**19**	**14**	**16**	35[9]
B[6] (mg/d)	**1.6**	**2.0**	1.3*	1.3*	100
Folate (µg/d)[8]	**180**	**200**	**400**	**400**	1,000[9]
B[12] (µg/d)	**2.0**	**2.0**	2.4*	2.4*	ND
Calcium (mg/d)	**800–1,200**	**800–1,200**[10]	1,000*	1,000*	2,500
Iron (mg/d)	**15**	**10**	**18**	**8**	45
Zinc (mg/d)	**12**	**15**	**8**	**11**	40

*AI: Adequate intakes are estimated when an RDA cannot be determined.

[†] UL: The maximum level of daily nutrient intake that is likely to pose no risk of adverse affects.

[1] Provitamin A carotenoids in the 1989 RDA were 1 µg vitamin A = 1 µg RE = 6 µg β-carotene = 12 µg α-carotene and β-cryptoxanthin. Provitamin A carotenoids in the 2001 DRI were 1 µg vitamin A =1µg RE = 12 µg β-carotene = 24 µg α-carotene and β-cryptoxanthin.

[2] For both men and women, the 1989 RDA for vitamin D was 10 µg/d for 19–24 year olds and 5 µg/d for 25 to 50 year olds.

[3] As α-tocopherol only.

[4] ULs for vitamin E include all forms of supplementary α-tocopherol.

[5] For vitamin K, the 1989 RDA for 19–24-year-old women and men was 60 & 70 µg/d, respectively; for 25–50-year-old women and men; it was 65 & 80 µg/d, respectively.

[6] ND: not determined. When a UL cannot be determined, extra caution may be warranted in consuming levels above the recommended intakes.

[7] As niacin equivalents (NE). 1 mg of niacin = 60 mg tryptophan.

[8] As dietary folate equivalents (DFE). 1 DFE = 1 µg food folate = 0.6 µg of folate from fortified food or as a supplement consumed with food = 0.5 µg of a supplement taken on an empty stomach.

[9] ULs for folate and niacin refer to forms supplied by supplements, fortified foods, or a combination of the two.

[10] For calcium, the 1989 RDA was 1,200 mg/day for 19–24-year-old men and women and 800 mg/d for 25–50-year-old men and women.

Reprinted from the International Food Information Council Foundation, Dietary Reference Intakes: An Update *(August 2002).*

Here is a checklist to help you decide if you should think about including an M/V in your plan. You may consider an M/V if these apply to you:

- I frequently skip meals.
- I have been consistently losing weight because I do not eat enough to support my physical activity needs.
- I have been told that I suffer from iron-deficiency anemia by my doctor.
- I eat a vegan diet (no animal products at all).
- I have been diagnosed with an eating disorder.

Antioxidants

They say . . .   Exercise is a stress on the body that increases your need for antioxidants.

Science says . . .   You may exercise to relieve mental or emotional stress. Ironically, one of the benefits of exercise is that it invokes physical stress. This physical stress, or stress on the muscles, cardiovascular system, respiratory function, and bone structure, is beneficial in the long run, as you become more conditioned and stronger. However, one of the consequences of this stress is muscle damage. The scientific jury is still out on whether antioxidants such as vitamin C, vitamin E, or flavonoids can help to reduce the damage or the subsequent soreness that accompanies it. It appears that there is a weak correlation between select antioxidants and muscle injury, but more research is warranted.

We say . . .   While the scientific evidence remains inconclusive, there is potential for benefit. If you choose to take an antioxidant supplement, mind your upper tolerable limits (see the table on page 145).

Caffeine

They say . . .   Caffeine helps you burn fat by protecting glycogen stores and can help you feel energized.

Science says . . .   Caffeine is definitely a mild stimulant commonly consumed by athletes in hope of improving performance. The expert consensus is that caffeine is a viable

> *Energy to Burn Nutritionism:* The average intake for those who drink coffee in the United States is two to four cups (200 to 400 mg of caffeine) each day.

ergogenic aid . . . but not because it promotes fat-burning or protects glycogen. Caffeine does increase the amount of fatty acids used during exercise, but it doesn't appear to spare glycogen. Furthermore, the result of using more fatty acids does not lead to weight loss, and the increase is not significant. It seems that the benefit is the impact it has on the central nervous system. As a stimulant, it can increase mental acuity and also may decrease your rating of perceived exertion—meaning you won't feel like you are working as hard as you may be.

We say . . . Moderate caffeine consumption is permitted by the NCAA and the IOC for athletes, so drink up . . . in moderation. Remember that some of you may not respond well to caffeine, however. Adverse effects reported included increases in blood pressure, gastrointestinal distress, an increase in heart rate, and insomnia. Pay attention to your response to caffeinated products, and if you're like me . . . coffee gives you a better personality . . . then enjoy two to four cups per day.

Caffeine has been scrutinized as a performance enhancer in the research and by the IOC and the NCAA. For those following the NCAA regulations, the 2007–2008 Banned Drug Classes note that caffeine is permitted as long as the athlete's urine concentration of caffeine remains below 15µg/mL. The IOC says that 12µg/mL is the cutoff. This allows athletes to take cold remedies if necessary and consume caffeinated beverages. This value equates to approximately 8 cups of percolated coffee or about 1,000 mg of caffeine for most people. Some folks may absorb the caffeine more rapidly and may find themselves approaching the peak level at 350 mg of caffeine. So be careful with your cup of coffee and drink it moderately for the benefits to your mood and personality rather than trying to chug a gallon for a mild performance boost. It could result in a higher urinary caffeine concentration and trouble.

Coffee is known to have varying levels of caffeine, and some beverages don't report how much they contain on their package, so some athletes try supplements. If you choose to use caffeine, stick to a moderate amount, somewhere in the order of 0.5 to 2 mg per pound of body weight (1 to 4 mg per kg of body weight).

> *Energy to Burn Nutritionism:* The Center for Science in the Public Interest (CSPI) reports that a Grande (16-oz) Starbucks Brewed Coffee contains about 320 mg of caffeine.

Creatine

They say . . . Creatine gives muscles energy to work harder and grow bigger.

Science says . . . Creatine is an amino acid that is naturally found in meat and fish, and is a stored form of energy for the muscles. The supplement creatine is packaged in powders, pills, sports bars, and liquids. In the body, creatine plays an important role in energy metabolism because it has a quick response and potential for buffering the acidic by-products of normal energy metabolism. Creatine gives you the energy you need for short bursts of activity. The reason the supplement came about is twofold: first, creatine, in the form of phosphocreatine, is stored only in small quantities; second, it supplies energy for only a short time . . . about ten to fifteen seconds . . . for maximal bouts of physical activity. In addition, creatine seems to increase the amount of water in your muscles and subsequently the amount of glycogen that can be stored.

Energy to Burn Nutritionism: Three hundred out of a thousand twelfth-grade football players surveyed said they used creatine to aid in recovery.

In research, an overview of all the studies shows that creatine is useful in the short term for increasing muscle when you perform repeated high-intensity, short-duration exercise, as well as helping you push harder. Creatine has been shown to be an effective supplement for:

- increasing lean body mass;
- gaining strength;
- improving recovery;
- enhancing endurance.

Creatine supplementation and exercise studies from 2007 provide nine points related to the use of creatine as a nutritional supplement, which constitute the position statement of the International Society of Sports Nutrition. The electronic version of this article is the complete one and can be found online at http://www.jissn.com/content/4/1/6.

1. Creatine monohydrate is the most effective ergogenic nutritional supplement currently available to athletes in terms of increasing high-intensity exercise capacity and lean body mass during training.

2. Creatine monohydrate supplementation is not only safe, but also possibly beneficial in regard to preventing injury and/or management of select medical conditions when taken within recommended guidelines.

3. There is no scientific evidence that the short- or long-term use of creatine monohydrate has any detrimental effects on otherwise healthy individuals.

4. If proper precautions and supervision are provided, supplementation in young athletes is acceptable and may provide a nutritional alternative to potentially dangerous anabolic drugs.

5. At present, creatine monohydrate is the most extensively studied and clinically effective form of creatine for use in nutritional supplements in terms of muscle uptake and ability to increase high-intensity exercise capacity.

6. The addition of carbohydrate or carbohydrate and protein to a creatine supplement appears to increase muscular retention of creatine, although the effect on performance measures may not be greater than using creatine monohydrate alone.

7. The quickest method of increasing muscle creatine stores appears to be to consume about 0.3 gram per kilogram per day of creatine monohydrate for at least three days followed by three to five grams per day thereafter to maintain elevated stores. Ingesting smaller amounts of creatine monohydrate (e.g., two to three grams per day) will increase muscle creatine stores over a three- to four-week period; however, the performance effects of this method of supplementation are less supported.

8. Creatine products are readily available as a dietary supplement and are regulated by the U.S. Food and Drug Administration (FDA). Specifically, in 1994, U.S. president Bill Clinton signed into law the Dietary Supplement Health and Education Act (DSHEA), which allows manufacturers/companies/brands to make structure-function claims; however, the law strictly prohibits disease claims for dietary supplements.

9. Creatine monohydrate has been reported to have a number of potentially beneficial uses in several clinical populations, and further research is warranted in these areas.

We say . . . Creatine has been shown to be safe and effective. Many athletes report an increase in muscle mass when they use creatine correctly with a resistance training program. However, everything can have side effects. Many athletes we have worked with complain that their muscles feel full of fluid and that they experience cramping. Results do vary, and not all athletes respond favorably to creatine. For young athletes, don't forget that studies have not looked into the effects creatine may have on your healthy growth process.

DHEA (Dehydroepiandrosterone)

They say . . . This prohormone will increase testosterone and therefore increase muscle mass.

Science says . . .   Yes, it's a precursor to testosterone and estrogen. But it's weak and the data say, don't bother. Science hasn't been able to show any benefit.

We say . . .   Need we say more? We will. All prohormones have been banned by the World Antidoping Agency.

Betaine

They say . . .   Betaine helps to improve muscle mass and strength.

Science says . . .   Betaine comes from natural foods such as beets, wheat germ, and spinach. It has been shown to be beneficial for sports performance and general health. Betaine donates methyl groups ($CH3$) needed for over one hundred different reactions essential for normal cell function, including synthesis of creatine, carnitine, and epinephrines. Research suggests that 2 to 3 grams per day is optimal for most athletes.

We say . . .   Preliminary research suggests that betaine may be useful in increasing strength and power when combined with resistance-type exercise and used in the proper amounts.

Beta-Alanine

They say . . .   It will increase muscle strength and delay fatigue.

Science says . . .   Beta-alanine has been known to act as a buffer in the muscle cells. As of late, it's been reviewed as a supplement to help manage the burning in the muscles that negatively affects performance during high-intensity exercise. On a cellular level, this "burning" is attributed to the acid production during intense exercise. Beta-alanine may help to decrease this performance prohibiter. A scientific review from the *Journal of Sports Sciences* points out that there may be benefits to buffering muscles during high-intensity exercise, but that the performance benefits and dosage recommendations still need investigation.

We say . . .   It looks promising for beta-alanine as a muscle buffer. The scientific review mentioned states that high doses may have side effects such as harmless tingling or mild flushing in the short term (subsiding in two hours), but that there aren't any long-term side effects noted in the research.

Chromium

They say . . .   It will make you lose weight!

Science says . . .   We eat chromium in many different foods . . . beef, poultry, eggs, nuts, and whole grains. It's an essential mineral and has become a popular dietary supplement over the years. Its role in the body is to make the body more sensitive to insulin and improve glucose utilization. When evaluated as an ergogenic aid, only one study, with football players, showed that chromium picolanate the supplement could increase muscle mass. Follow-up studies revealed that this supplement did not provide any benefit for muscle gains or any changes in body composition.

We say . . . Take it off your list. Not only does chromium picolanate lack the science to support its use, there also may be side effects. In animal studies, chronic use was associated with chromosomal damage. The bottom line: no benefits identified, only potential for ill effects . . . therefore, waste of money.

The Bulk of Ergo Aids

There seems to be an endless supply of ergogenic aids available for sport and dietary supplements available for weight loss. In addition to those already discussed, here are some others you might encounter, along with what the scientific literature has to say. Our recommendations are in the right column.

Aid	Question	Science Says . . .	We Say . . .
Carnitine: made from amino acids lysine, and methionine.	Does it increase fat use?	Nearly all studies failed to find a benefit to increasing fat use.	The science isn't there yet. A couple of studies found benefits for exercise, but it's too soon to supplement. . . . Back to the lab.
Coenzyme Q10, aka Ubiquinone: found in all cells in the mitochondria (our energy station).	Does it increase aerobic capacity?	Very little in the way of athletic performance improvements; may have antioxidant potential.	Insufficient data to call it a performance enhancer. May have antioxidant potential and should be investigated further for that benefit.
Glutamine: nonessential amino acid.	Does it increase protein synthesis and limit synthesis, breakdown? Does it help with immune and gut health?	Although amino acids are helpful for protein glutamine alone doesn't seem to provide additional benefit.	It appears to be safe, but it doesn't seem to have special benefits for protein synthesis or breakdown prevention. Additionally, may help with immune and gut health.
Medium Chain Triglycerides (MCT): fatty acids that are released during normal fat digestion.	Does it increase fat oxidation during long-duration exercise?	MCTs will be used during exercise, but they don't appear to make a big difference on their own.	Sure, it's a fuel source, but the evidence that it's an ergogenic aid is lacking.

Above and Beyond: Functional Foods

We know that food serves many functions: it provides the nutrients we need to do work and gives us energy (again to do work), the ability to maintain, repair, and rebuild our body, fuel a workout or workday, and something to do when we get together with friends and family. What about above and beyond these everyday necessities? According to the International Food Information Council (IFIC), there are foods and ingredients that may provide a health benefit beyond (and above) basic nutrition. IFIC has compiled a thorough table of functional food components, food sources, and their potential benefits.

EXAMPLES OF FUNCTIONAL COMPONENTS*

Class/Components	Source*	Potential Benefits
Carotenoids		
Beta-carotene	Carrots, pumpkin, sweet potato, cantaloupe	Neutralizes free radicals, which may damage cells; bolsters cellular antioxidant defenses; can be made into vitamin A in the body
Lutein, zeaxanthin	Kale, collards, spinach, corn, eggs, citrus	May contribute to maintenance of healthy vision
Lycopene	Tomatoes and processed tomato products, watermelon, red/pink grapefruit	May contribute to maintenance of prostate health
Dietary (functional and total) Fiber		
Insoluble fiber	Wheat bran, corn bran, fruit skins	May contribute to maintenance of a healthy digestive tract; may reduce the risk of some types of cancer
Beta glucan**	Oat bran, oatmeal, oat flour, barley, rye	May reduce risk of coronary heart disease (CHD)
Soluble fiber**	Psyllium seed husk, peas, beans, apples, citrus fruit	May reduce risk of CHD and some types of cancer
Whole grains**	Cereal grains, whole wheat bread, oatmeal, brown rice	May reduce risk of CHD and some types of cancer; may contribute to maintenance of healthy blood glucose levels
Fatty Acids		
Monounsaturated fatty acids (MUFAs)**	Tree nuts, olive oil, canola oil	May reduce risk of CHD

Class/Components	Source*	Potential Benefits
Polyunsaturated fatty acids (PUFAs)— omega-3 fatty acids—ALA	Walnuts, flax	May contribute to maintenance of heart health; may contribute to maintenance of mental and visual function
PUFAs—omega-3 fatty acids— DHA/EPA**	Salmon, tuna, marine, and other fish oils	May reduce risk of CHD; may contribute to maintenance of mental and visual function
Conjugated linoleic acid (CLA)	Beef and lamb; some cheese	May contribute to maintenance of desirable body composition and healthy immune function
Flavonoids		
Anthocyanins— cyanidin, delphini- din, malvidin	Berries, cherries, red grapes	Bolster cellular antioxidant defenses; may contribute to maintenance of brain function
Flavanols— catechins, epicatechins, epigallocatechin, procyanidins	Tea, cocoa, chocolate, apples, grapes	May contribute to maintenance of heart health
Flavanones— hesperetin, naringenin	Citrus foods	Neutralize free radicals, which may damage cells; bolster cellular antioxidant defenses
Flavonols— quercetin, kaempf- erol, isorhamnetin, myricetin	Onions, apples, tea, broccoli	Neutralize free radicals, which may damage cells; bolster cellular antioxidant defenses
Proanthocyanidins	Cranberries, cocoa, apples, strawberries, grapes, wine, peanuts, cinnamon	May contribute to maintenance of urinary tract health and heart health
Isothiocyanates		
Sulforaphane	Cauliflower, broccoli, broccoli sprouts, cabbage, kale, horseradish	May enhance detoxification of undesirable compounds; bolsters cellular antioxidant defenses
Minerals		
Calcium**	Sardines, spinach, yogurt, low-fat dairy products, fortified foods and beverages	May reduce the risk of osteoporosis
Magnesium	Spinach, pumpkin seeds, whole-grain breads and cereals, halibut, Brazil nuts	May contribute to maintenance of normal muscle and nerve function, healthy immune function, and bone health
Potassium**	Potatoes, low-fat dairy products, whole-grain breads and cereals, citrus juices, beans, bananas	May reduce the risk of high blood pressure and stroke, in combination with a low-sodium diet

(continued)

Class/Components	Source*	Potential Benefits
Selenium	Fish, red meat, grains, garlic, liver, eggs	Neutralizes free radicals, which may damage cells; may contribute to healthy immune function
Phenolic Acids		
Caffeic acid, Ferulic acid	Apples, pears, citrus fruits, some vegetables, coffee	May bolster cellular antioxidant defenses; may contribute to maintenance of healthy vision and heart health
Plant Stanols/Sterols		
Free Stanols/sterols**	Corn, soy, wheat, wood oils, fortified foods and beverages	May reduce risk of CHD
Stanol/sterol esters**	Fortified table spreads, stanol ester dietary supplements	May reduce risk of CHD
Polyols		
Sugar alcohols**— xylitol, sorbitol, mannitol, lactitol	Some chewing gums and other food	Applications may reduce risk of dental caries
Prebiotics		
Inulin, fructo-oligosaccharides (FOS), polydextrose	Whole grains, onions, some fruits, garlic, honey, leeks, fortified foods and beverages	May improve gastrointestinal health; may improve calcium absorption
Probiotics		
Yeast, lactobacilli, bifidobacteria, and other specific strains of beneficial bacteria	Certain yogurts and other cultured dairy and non-dairy applications	May improve gastrointestinal health and systemic immunity; benefits are strain-specific
Phytoestrogens		
Isoflavones— daidzein, genistein	Soybeans and soy-based foods	May contribute to maintenance of bone health, healthy brain and immune function; for women, may contribute to maintenance of menopausal health
Lignans	Flax, rye, some vegetables	May contribute to maintenance of heart health and healthy immune function
Soy Protein		
Soy protein**	Soybeans and soy-based foods	May reduce risk of CHD
Sulfides/Thiols		
Diallyl sulfide, Allyl methyl trisulfide	Garlic, onions, leeks, scallions	May enhance detoxification of undesirable compounds; may contribute to maintenance of heart health and healthy immune function

Class/Components	Source*	Potential Benefits
Dithiolthiones	Cruciferous vegetables	May enhance detoxification of undesirable compounds; may contribute to maintenance of healthy immune function
Vitamins		
A***	Organ meats, milk, eggs, carrots, sweet potatoes, spinach	May contribute to maintenance of healthy vision, immune function, and bone health; may contribute to cell integrity
B_1 (thiamin)	Lentils, peas, long-grain brown rice, Brazil nuts	May contribute to maintenance of mental function; helps regulate metabolism
B_2 (riboflavin)	Lean meats, eggs, green leafy vegetables	Helps support cell growth; helps regulate metabolism
B_3 (niacin)	Dairy products, poultry, fish, nuts, eggs	Helps support cell growth; helps regulate metabolism
B_5 (pantothenic acid)	Organ meats, lobster, soybeans, lentils	Helps regulate metabolism and hormone synthesis
B_6 (pyridoxine)	Beans, nuts, legumes, fish, meat, whole grains	May contribute to maintenance of healthy immune function; helps regulate metabolism
B_9 (folate)**	Beans, legumes, citrus foods, green leafy vegetables, fortified breads and cereals	May reduce a woman's risk of having a child with a brain or spinal cord defect
B_{12} (cobalamin)	Eggs, meat, poultry, milk	May contribute to maintenance of mental function; helps regulate metabolism and supports blood cell formation
Biotin	Liver, salmon, dairy, eggs, oysters	Helps regulate metabolism and hormone synthesis
C	Guava, sweet red/green pepper, kiwi, citrus fruit, strawberries	Neutralizes free radicals, which may damage cells; may contribute to maintenance of bone health and immune function
D	Sunlight, fish, fortified milk and cereals	Helps regulate calcium and phosphorus; helps contribute to bone health; may contribute to healthy immune function; helps support cell growth
E	Sunflower seeds, almonds, hazelnuts, turnip greens	Neutralizes free radicals, which may damage cells; may contribute to healthy immune function and maintenance of heart health

* Examples are not an all-inclusive list.
** FDA-approved health claim established for component.
*** Preformed vitamin A is found in foods that come from animals. Provitamin A carotenoids are found in many darkly colored fruits and vegetables and are a major source of vitamin A for vegetarians.

Reprinted from the International Food Information Council Foundation, Functional Food Backgrounder *(November 2006).*

Printed in the 2007–2009 IFIC Foundation Media Guide on Food Safety and Nutrition.

Who Makes the Rules for Functional Foods?

As the popularity of the term "functional food" has grown, the FDA has decided to get involved to make sure that every food package doesn't start making claims about its special qualities without adequate evidence. In 1990, the FDA approved the use of health claims on food labels so consumers could identify which foods had additional functions. Based on the Nutrition Labeling and Education Act, foods and their components can bear a health claim that describes the relationship between the food (or component) and a disease risk or illness if the science supports it.

A food company can petition for a health claim to be considered for their package based on the breadth and extent of the research available. In addition, beginning in 1997, the FDA Modernization Act (FDAMA) grants manufacturers the right to expedite the process for using health claims if the claim is based on up- to-date, published, authoritative statements by federal scientific bodies (ADA Position 2004). Examples of the authorized organizations include the National Academy of Science, National Institutes for Health (NIH), and the Centers for Disease Control and Prevention. Therefore, if the NIH gives a food and disease link, manufacturers can receive approval more quickly (120 days).

There are five types of health-related claims that you may see on the food you buy. Once authorized, the following are FDA-permitted claims on a food or dietary supplement.

A food label can:

- Say that a product contains a certain amount of a particular nutrient. For example, the label can read that a certain amount of a functional food component is present in the food.
- Give a description of the effect the product has on normal body processes.
- Provide the health benefits of a particular category of foods, such as with fruits and vegetables.
- Report a preapproved developing link between a food and the risk of disease.
- Report a preapproved connection between a food and the risk of disease or illness.

The Ultimate in Functional Foods: Fruits and Vegetables

Looking for the ultimate in functional foods? Look no farther than your produce aisle or local farm stand. They may not be on every commercial or come in a clever, man-made package, but they are the quintessential functional foods. Manufacturers may try, but fruits and vegetables represent the truly "natural" health food. Fruits and vegetables pack in the nutrients while remaining light in calories. Loaded with antioxidants, phytochemicals, and physiologically active components that protect us from illness and promote health, fruits and vegetables are superstars. Individual stars include tomato products as rich sources of the cancer-risk reducer lycopene, broccoli's famed association with reducing risk of certain cancers, and berries' ability to boost antioxidant defenses. On the whole, fruits and vegetables have been shown to shine by cutting a fruit and veggie enthusiast's cancer risk in half compared to their produce naysayers.

Fit Nutrition: A Vitamin and Mineral Handbook

When we talk to athletes about vitamins and minerals, many believe that these nutrients give them energy or build muscle (they don't); aid recovery (some may); help heal an injury (maybe); or in the supplement form, make up for a bad diet (good try). We want to emphasize that vitamins and minerals are important and play a role in a high-energy eating plan—with a balanced diet, it's likely that you will get all the vitamins and minerals you need. We think it's important to manage expectations and give the bottom line on what they can and cannot deliver—emphasizing that unless you're deficient, extra vitamins and minerals will not enhance your performance.

Food First, Supplements Second

Vitamins and minerals are referred to as *micronutrients*, because we need them in tiny or micro amounts in our diet compared to *macronutrients*, which are proteins, carbohydrates, and fats, which are needed in larger or macro quantities in our diet. Although we don't require gobs of vitamins and minerals, thirty-five of them (thirteen vitamins and twenty-two minerals) are considered essential for life. However, new bioactive substances are constantly being isolated, and most nutritionists believe that other essential nutrients will soon be identified.

Vitamins and minerals are necessary for virtually every body process, whether it's flexing a muscle, maintaining blood pressure, or absorbing calcium from milk or broccoli. They are also needed for a number of reactions specific to energy metabolism, getting oxygen shuttled around the body, and growing and repairing muscle tissue.

As dietitians and sports nutritionists, we believe the best advice is "food first, supplements second" and that supplements cannot make up for an unbalanced diet. They are best when they are used to supplement a healthy, balanced diet.

Use this section to see the most important vitamins and minerals that most of us are likely to eat inadequate amounts of. We'll tell you why you need them, how much you need, and how to ensure that you're getting the right amount . . . and not too much. See pages 168–170 for a table of how much you need and where to find the vitamins and minerals your body requires.

Vitamin and Minerals at a Glance

Fat-soluble vitamins include A, D, E, and K, while vitamin C and the B vitamins are water-soluble. We need only tiny amounts of vitamins in our diet. In fact, in a year, you need less than a pound of vitamins compared to the two thousand pounds of food we eat. But even they are essential for life, as our bodies cannot manufacture vitamins and minerals.

Most vitamins play some role in muscle contractions or the ability to convert food into energy and in energy metabolism. Several B vitamins are necessary for storing excess calories as fat; breaking down glycogen into glucose; aerobic metabolism (oxidative metabolism); and the digestion and absorption of nutrients. Folic acid and B_{12} also are necessary for red blood cell development; without enough, anemia can result.

Water-Soluble Vitamins

Vitamin B_1 (Thiamine)
Required for energy, the production of branched-chain amino acids, and carbohydrate metabolism, it is thought that B_1 requirements may be slightly higher for individuals who have high energy expenditures. Overall, however, physical activity does not appear to significantly increase the body's requirement for thiamine. But for those engaged in intense training, higher levels of intake may be required. However, of the few studies conducted with athletes supplemented with thiamine, none has found conclusive evidence that exceeding the RDA value for B_1 provides a performance benefit.

Vitamin B_2 (Riboflavin)
Riboflavin is involved in metabolic reactions for energy production. While there are no data to suggest that athletes need more than the RDA of

riboflavin in their diet for optimal performance, research does suggest that riboflavin requirements may be higher for athletes than for the general population.

Niacin

Niacin is actually a family of molecules that also includes nicotinic acid and nicotinamide. The B vitamin is needed for glucose metabolism and energy production. Either too much or too little can be detrimental to performance. A deficiency can affect glycolysis and the oxidation process affecting both anaerobic- and aerobic-type performance. At high doses it may shift metabolism to utilize carbohydrate and decrease free fatty acids, potentially impairing endurance performance. The requirement for niacin is usually linked to energy intake, which means that athletes who have high energy intakes will have a proportionately higher need for niacin. Overall, there is no evidence to support higher amounts of niacin above the RDA for a performance benefit.

Vitamin B_6 (Pyridoxine)

Also referred to as pyridoxal, this B vitamin is essential for about a hundred reactions in the body, including the production and metabolism of carbohydrates, fats, and proteins. It also is involved in the manufacture of compounds necessary for hemoglobin, the compound that carries oxygen through the bloodstream. While some initial studies suggested that endurance athletes may have increased needs for B_6, more recent data suggest that the RDA is adequate.

Vitamin B_{12} (Cyanocobalamin)

This B vitamin is necessary for DNA synthesis and for the formation and function of red blood cells; deficiencies can lead to anemia. Because of its role in oxygen-bearing red blood cells, it has been suggested that additional B_{12} might improve performance in athletic events in which oxidative metabolism is important. However, there is no evidence that B_{12} supplements or injections improve performance. And B_{12} deficiency among athletes is rare. Since B_{12} is found only in animal-based products, vegan athletes need to take B_{12} supplements or include B_{12}-fortified foods in their diets. Supplementing with large doses of other vitamins, such as vitamin C, may actually decrease vitamin B_{12} availability and lead to a B_{12} deficiency.

Folate (Folacin, folic acid)

This B vitamin is also involved in DNA synthesis and the formation of amino acids and is important during times of growth and development. A deficiency of this nutrient can lead to anemia. Recent Centers for Disease Control and Prevention data have shown that a growing percentage of women in the United States have deficient blood folate levels. However, there is no evidence that in the absence of a deficiency, supplemental folate can improve athletic performance. Athletes should strive to meet the RDA for folate.

Pantothenic Acid

Pantothenic acid is necessary for energy production from proteins, carbohydrates, and fats. Few studies have been conducted to determine if athletes have increased requirements for pantothenic acid. For optimal performance, athletes should strive to meet the AI for pantothenic acid. Pantothenic acid is present in virtually all plant and animal foods, so inadequate intake is rare.

Biotin

This vitamin serves as a coenzyme in many metabolic reactions and is essential for carbohydrate, fat, and amino acid metabolism. Biotin is needed in energy production, suggesting that inadequate intake could affect performance, but to date, no studies have been conducted to determine if athletes require additional biotin above the AI level.

Vitamin C (Ascorbic acid, ascorbate)

This antioxidant vitamin is necessary for collagen synthesis, breaking down fatty acids, and forming neurotransmitters in the brain and nervous system. There are data to suggest that vitamin C helps protect against upper respiratory tract infections (URTIs) or common colds among endurance and ultraendurance athletes.

Athletes competing and training in ultraendurance events may benefit from taking five hundred milligrams a day of vitamin C, and those in other nonendurance activities may benefit from at least a hundred grams a day. There is no evidence that doses at higher amounts will provide additional benefits, and they may have adverse effects.

Fat-Soluble Vitamins

Vitamin A (Retinol) and Beta-carotene

This antioxidant vitamin is best known for its role in maintaining healthy vision, but it is also needed for reproduction and bone formation. Beta-carotene serves as a precursor to vitamin A, meaning that when the body needs vitamin A, it will convert beta-carotene into vitamin A. Beta-

carotene is just one of the hundreds of carotenoids that have been identified, including lutein and lycopene.

Carotenoids are also antoxidants and are thought to have potential
anti-cancer activity when consumed in foods, but supplements appear to
be less helpful and in some cases have been found to be potentially harmful. There is some evidence that supplemental beta-carotene may have
adverse effects on lung tissue, so it is not recommended that athletes supplement their diets with beta-carotene unless suggested by a health care
professional.

There is no evidence to suggest that athletes should consume more than
the RDA for vitamin A or beta-carotene. Since vitamin A is stored in the
body, it can have negative health effects. Studies show that excessive
amounts can reduce bone-mineral density, among other negative effects.

Vitamin D

This hormone/vitamin is unique in that the body can generally manufacture enough on its own if the skin is exposed to adequate sunlight. Vitamin
D is essential for calcium metabolism and bone health. Emerging research
shows it to be involved in a much wider spectrum of body functions, from
helping prevent certain types of cancer and type 2 diabetes. However,
there has been little research to investigate the effects of physical activity on vitamin D requirements or the effects of vitamin D on exercise performance. While there is no evidence that athletes are at special risk for
vitamin D deficiency or that they need additional vitamin D, it is important for athletes in weight-sensitive sports (gymnasts, distance runners,
and cyclists) to take adequate vitamin D to help maintain healthy bones.
In recent years, as Americans have become more aware of the harmful
effects of UV rays from sunlight, vitamin D status has declined. By blocking the sun's UV rays, sunscreens are blocking the trigger that allows the
body to manufacture vitamin D.

More recent research has linked diets rich in vitamin D to a reduced
risk for certain cancers, diabetes, and overall death rates. Most of the
research on vitamin D has occurred in the past five years, and it is thought
that the current recommendation of 400 IU per day used on food labels
as the daily value may be too low; four to six times that amount may be
optimal. While it's too early to recommend vitamin D as a preventive
measure against disease, ensuring that you have foods that contain vitamin D in your diet is essential. Only a few foods naturally contain vitamin
D, and only dairy products and a few 100 percent fruit juices are fortified

with the nutrient. In addition, expose your skin to sunshine for small, safe amounts of time to manufacture the nutrient. Spending 15 minutes in the summer sun can enable the body to produce 15,000 IU of vitamin D or more than thirty-seven times the RDI of 400 IU.

Vitamin E (Tocopherols, Tocotrienols)
Vitamin E is actually a family of eight compounds known as tocopherols and tocotrienols. As an antioxidant, vitamin E helps to protect cell membranes from oxidative damage and is known to help protect the immune system. Vitamin E has long been thought to possess cardioprotective qualities, but recent research on vitamin E supplements and heart disease has been less conclusive.

Several studies of marathon runners have evaluated the effects of vitamin E supplementation before marathons or other ultraendurance events, such as the Marathon des Sables, a six-stage running event across the Sahara. French researchers randomly assigned runners to either an antioxidant group, who took twenty-four milligrams of vitamin E (along with vitamin C and beta-carotene) daily for three weeks before the event, or to a control group. Blood was taken from the athletes two days prior to the race, after the third stage, then again at the end. The researchers found that athletes who took the supplement did not have elevated TBARS (a measure of oxidative stress) compared to the control subjects, who exhibited elevated TBARs during the race.

Other studies have found similar results. Because vitamin E protects muscle from free radical damage, it has potential as an ergogenic aid for athletes. However, research suggests it holds more promise as a way to prevent oxidative damage as a result of exercise, rather than actually improving exercise performance. There is no conclusive data to suggest that vitamin E acts as a performance enhancer, but since many athletes don't get enough of this nutrient, it's important to pay close attention to the level of E in your diet or to consider a supplement containing vitamin E.

Vitamin K
Vitamin K is the fat-soluble nutrient best known for blood clotting. What's less known is that vitamin K is also required for the formation of osteocalcin, a compound necessary for optimal bone growth and density. Deficiencies of vitamin K may be more common than previously thought due to diets high in refined carbohydrates and megadoses of vitamins A and E. Antibiotics also can impair vitamin K status by decreasing intestinal bacterial function responsible for the production of vitamin K.

Athletes at risk for low bone density and bone mass may need additional vitamin K in their diets over and above the current AI.

Major Minerals

Minerals are inorganic compounds classified by the amount required in the body: macrominerals are required in amounts ranging from hundreds to thousands of milligrams, while trace minerals are required in amounts of only a few milligrams or even micrograms. Sodium, potassium, calcium, phosphorus, and magnesium are macrominerals, while iron, zinc, selenium, and others are trace minerals.

Sodium, Potassium, and Chloride

Sodium, potassium, and chloride are the three major electrolytes in the body that maintain electrical signaling between the outside and the inside of every cell in the body. Sodium and chloride are in the fluid outside of the cells, in the extracellular fluid, while potassium is in the intracellular fluid. They are involved with maintaining fluid balance, nerve transmission, and muscle contractions.

Sweating increases the need for sodium because the average sodium loss ranges from 460 to 1,840 mg of sodium per liter of sweat and can only get worse in the heat.

Exercise-induced low-plasma sodium, also called hyponatremia (sodium concentration of <130 mmol/l, normal range 135 to 146 mmol/l), has been observed with increasing frequency during the past decade, with reports of up to nearly 30 percent of endurance athletes being affected. Hyponatremia has been reported in many endurance athletes, from marathoners to Ironman competitors, and is thought to occur when athletes become dehydrated and drink water only without additional sources of sodium (i.e., sports drinks, bars, or gels).

Most athletes get enough sodium, potassium, and chloride in their diets as they eat more calories and naturally get more salt (sodium chloride) in their diets than do nonathletes. However, endurance athletes need to pay special attention to their sodium and chloride intake before, during, and after training and racing to ensure that they are replenishing what is lost in sweat.

For the endurance athletes, loss of fluid and sodium can affect performance because of the dreaded heat cramps—which seem to be different from cramps due to fatigue. Fatigue cramps are localized muscle cramps related to being too tired or working too hard. The best remedy for these cramps is stretching, icing, and massaging. Heat cramps, on the other hand, occur during prolonged exercise in hot conditions and may have more to do with large losses of fluid and sodium due to heavy sweating. Endurance athletes tend to be heavy sweaters who lose large amount of sodium through sweat.

Electrolytes Lost in Sweat
Sodium: 40–80 mmol/L or 920–1840 mg/L
Chloride: 30–70 mmol/L or 1062–2478 mg/L
Potassium: 4–8 mmol/L or 156–312 mg/L
Calcium: 3–4 mmol/L or 120–160 mg/L
Magnesium: 1–4 mmol/L or 24–96 mg/L

Average Amounts of Electrolytes Lost in 1 Liter (33.8 ounces) of Sweat
Sodium: 1,380 mg
Chloride: 1,770 mg
Potassium: 234 mg
Calcium: 140 mg
Magnesium: 60 mg

Calcium
Calcium is the most abundant element in the body. We have a few pounds of it in our body at any given time, with 99 percent of the body's calcium providing structure to our bones and teeth, with the remainder in our blood, body fluids, muscles, and other soft tissues. The mineral is necessary for bone metabolism, blood, neuromuscular function, muscle contractions, cell membranes, and hundreds of other reactions in the body.

Calcium is often lacking in athletes' diets, and some evidence suggests that athletes who sweat a lot in the heat may have additional calcium losses in sweat and may need more than the AI for calcium in their diets; a calcium supplement may be needed. Keep in mind that the efficiency of absorption of calcium from supplements is greatest when calcium is taken in doses of no more than five hundred milligrams at a time.

Phosphorus
As the second most abundant mineral in the body, 85 percent is in our bones and teeth, and the remaining 15 percent help with many other functions, including energy production. Phosphorus is in muscles as part of the high-energy compounds phosphocreatine and adenosine triphos-

phate (ATP). ATP is the supplier of energy for muscle contractions. Phosphorus also is involved in buffering of the acid end products of energy metabolism, which is why you may have heard of phosphate-loading. This was a technique designed to buffer lactic acid buildup but was found not to provide performance-enhancing benefits.

While phosphorus is essential for healthy bones, too much of the nutrient actually weakens bones. High phosphorus intakes can decrease vitamin D production, affecting calcium absorption. Phosphorus is in many foods in the diet, so overconsumption is more of an issue for athletes than not getting enough of the nutrient. Drinking too many carbonated beverages, which are high in phosphorus, can increase risk of bone fractures. There is no evidence to support getting more than the RDA for phosphorus for active individuals.

Magnesium

Magnesium is a mineral essential for energy production and is involved as a cofactor in more than three hundred enzyme systems in the body. It also is needed to manufacture glycogen, the storage form of blood glucose in the muscles and liver. In addition, it works with calcium and phosphorus to maintain bone health. In fact, 60 to 65 percent of the body's magnesium is in bone. Magnesium also works in conjunction with sodium and potassium to maintain blood pressure.

Of the studies conducted on magnesium supplementation with athletes, there is inconclusive evidence that the nutrient acts as a performance enhancer. However, studies show that loss of magnesium in the urine and sweat is higher in people who exercise, especially in hot conditions. Obtaining the RDA for the nutrient is considered adequate.

Iron

Iron is key for athletes because it is needed to form hemoglobin in red blood cells and myoglobin in muscle. Iron helps increase the oxygen-carrying capacity of blood, which is critical for muscles to extract oxygen for energy production. In addition to supplying oxygen to cells, iron helps facilitate energy transfer within cells. Training, regardless of the type, increases iron requirements due to increased iron turnover in tissues, iron losses in sweat, and the breakdown of red blood cells during training.

Many athletes—especially female athletes, runners, and vegetarians—are at risk for low iron, which will result in a reduced amount of hemoglobin in the blood. In fact, iron depletion is relatively common among athletes, and as a result, it has been suggested that athletes need much more than the

RDA for iron. Some have recommended seventeen to eighteen milligrams per day for men and twenty-three milligrams per day for women who are menstruating. Some studies have found that as many as 60 percent of female athletes may be at risk for anemia. For those identified as anemic, a doctor may recommend up to one hundred milligrams of iron per day—at this level, you need to have a doctor prescribe it; don't do this on your own.

Iron-deficiency anemia causes loss of appetite, fatigue, sluggishness, and a high rate of perceived exertion when working out. Endurance athletes, vegetarians, and females should have their iron levels and hematocrit levels checked annually or twice a year to detect if iron levels are sufficient. Ferritin is the storage form of iron, while hematocrit is a measurement of red blood cells, which carry iron. As the iron supply decreases, the serum iron concentration falls, and the saturation of transferrin (the amount of iron it stores) is decreased. Though no single test tells the whole story, low hematocrit and low hemoglobin together typically signal anemia. Low serum ferritin with normal hemoglobin suggest early-stage iron deficiency (borderline anemia).

Iron supplements are commonly used among athletes. If you have low iron, it's almost impossible to reverse in a timely fashion (fewer than one to two years) without supplementation. Taking an iron supplement daily can help improve anemia in about three months. Since excess iron can be toxic for people who suffer from hemochromatosis or iron overload, it is best to have your blood levels of iron checked frequently to ensure that you are not at risk for iron overload.

Signs of Iron Deficiency
- Pale skin
- Elevated resting heart rate
- Feeling run-down
- Weakness or lethargy
- Lack of motivation
- Mood changes
- Loss of appetite

For those striving to get more iron, it's important to know that only about 10 percent of the iron you eat is absorbed. And what you eat or drink can further diminish how much iron your body absorbs. Heme iron, or iron from animal foods, has the highest absorption and is affected little by dietary factors. For best absorption of other foods and supplements, consume iron supplements or iron-containing plant foods with a vitamin C source and avoid phytate- or polyphenol-rich options at about the time you have an iron-rich meal or supplement.

Iron enhancers include vitamin C–containing foods such as citrus fruit and juices that enhance iron absorption. Several compounds in foods inhibit iron absorption: phytate in whole grains, wheat bran, wheat germ, seeds, soy, oatmeal, and lentils; polyphenols (tannins) in tea, red wine, cocoa, and coffee; excess intake of other minerals (zinc, calcium, magnesium); oxalates from spinach, rhubarb, Swiss chard, and dark chocolate; and excess use of antacids.

Zinc

Zinc is ubiquitous in our bodies; about 60 percent of the mineral is in muscle, 29 percent in bone, and the remainder in the GI tract, skin, kidneys, and other major organs. Zinc has a role in more than three hundred reactions in the body, is associated with keeping the immune system healthy, and is involved in gene expression. Zinc also affects metabolic rate, thyroid hormones, protein utilization, and glycogen storage.

Zinc is lost through urine and sweat. However, consumption of the RDA appears to be enough for athletes; zinc status has not been found to be negatively affected by exercise training when zinc intake is adequate, and additional zinc will not provide a performance-enhancing benefit. However, athletes maintaining low body weights, such as wrestlers, dancers, and gymnasts, may not meet their zinc requirements. And the zinc requirement for strict vegetarians may be as much as 50 percent greater than for nonvegetarians.

Selenium

This antioxidant nutrient is essential for normal immune system and thyroid hormones, and some research suggests it has anticancer properties. Selenium supplements have been studied for endurance athletes to see if selenium reduces oxidative damage. However, research does not support the need for selenium in the diet above the RDA.

Chromium

Chromium is involved in carbohydrate, fat, and protein metabolism. Chromium is thought to stimulate insulin and therefore increase protein synthesis in muscle and help regulate blood sugar. At health food stores, chromium is often sold as chromium picolinate, a highly absorbable form of chromium, and marketed to increase lean body mass. However, studies have found mixed results; overall there appears to be some benefit for strength- or power-focused athletes but little or no benefit for endurance athletes.

How Much Do I Need? Where Do I Get It?

Following is a chart of the dietary reference intakes (DRIs), which explains how much of a specific nutrient is needed daily.

Nutrient	What It Does	Male RDA or AI*	Female RDA or AI	Best Sources	Adverse Effects of Excessive Amounts
Fat-Soluble Vitamins					
Vitamin A	Maintains vision; strengthens immune system; act as antioxidant	900 mcg	700 mcg	Carrots; pumpkins; sweet potatoes; mangoes; spinach and dark, leafy greens; liver; dairy products; seafood	Headache, vomiting; bone loss; peeling of skin; liver toxicity; may cause birth defects in pregnant women (only vitamin A, not beta-carotene)
Vitamin D	Aids in the absorption and regulation of calcium and phos-phorus necessary for strong bones and teeth; may play a role in fat metabolism	5 mcg/ 200IU	5 mcg/ 200IU	Fortified milk, and dairy-fortified cereals; cod-liver oil; oysters; fish; eggs	May increase calcium to unhealthy levels in blood
Vitamin E	Acts as an antioxidant to help protect cells from free radicals	15 mg	15 mg	Vegetable oils, whole grains, wheat germ, nuts and seeds; vegetables	May impair blood clotting
Vitamin K	Necessary for blood clotting, bone formation; helps regulate calcium	120 mcg	90 mcg	Leafy, green vegetables; plant oils and margarine; broccoli, peas, green beans	No adverse effects, can counteract the the effects of blood-thinning drugs such as Coumadin
Water-Soluble Vitamins					
Thiamin (vitamin B_1)	Necessary to metabolize carbohydrates and amino acids	1.2 mg	1.1 mg	Enriched grains and cereals; whole grains; fortified cereals	No adverse effects reported
Riboflavin	Necessary for con-verting carbohydrates, proteins, and fats into energy; essential for the production of red blood cells; maintains healthy skin and eyes	1.3 mg	1.1 mg	Almonds; brewer's yeast; milk, yogurt; fortified breads and cereals; wheat germ	No adverse effects reported

Nutrient	What It Does	Male RDA or AI*	Female RDA or AI	Best Sources	Adverse Effects of Excessive Amounts
Vitamin B$_6$	Needed to metabolize protein and carbohydrates; essential for brain and the production of red blood cells	1.3 mg	1.3 mg	Meat, fish, poultry; eggs; beans; whole grains; seeds; oysters	No adverse effects reported
Vitamin B$_{12}$	Aids in red blood cell formation; helps build and maintain central nervous system	2.4 mcg	2.4 mcg	Clams; meats; oysters; fish; yogurt, milk, and cheese; eggs; fortified breakfast cereals	No adverse effects reported
Niacin	Required for energy metabolism to convert carbohydrates, proteins, and fats into usable energy; nicotinic acid form lowers cholesterol	16 mg	14 mg	Meats; fish; poultry; peanuts and peanut butter; beef; enriched grain products (cereals and breads)	Gastrointestinal distress, flushing of face and neck in large doses
Folate/ Folic acid	Builds DNA and RNA, the building blocks of all cells; prevents some birth defects; lowers homocysteine levels, thereby protecting the heart	400 mcg	400 mcg	Enriched grains; dark, leafy greens; whole grains; fortified breads, flours, and cereals; citrus	Masks vitamin B$_{12}$ deficiency
Vitamin C	Acts as an antioxidant to help protect cells from free radical damage; essential for collagen formation and wound healing; enhances iron absorption	90 mg	75 mg	Fruits and vegetables	Gastrointestinal distress, kidney stones, excess iron absorption
Pantothenic acid	Protein, carbohydrate, and fat metabolism	5 mg	5 mg	Poultry, seafood, nuts, seeds, avocados, whole grains	None reported
Biotin	Functions as a coenzyme in many metabolic reactions in the body	30 mcg	30 mcg	Nuts, eggs, soybeans, fish	None reported
Minerals					
Sodium	Body water balance; acid-base balance, nerve transmission	1,500 mg	1,500 mg	Table salt, processed foods	Hypertension in salt-sensitive
Potassium	Body water balance; acid-base balance, nerve transmission	4,700 mg	4,700 mg	Fruits, vegetables, dairy products, nuts	Heart problems
Chloride	Body water balance; acid-base balance, nerve transmission	2,300 mg	2,300 mg	Table salt; processed foods	Elevated blood pressure

(continued)

(continued)

Nutrient	What It Does	Male RDA or AI*	Female RDA or AI	Best Sources	Adverse Effects of Excessive Amounts
Phosphorus	Bone and teeth, acid-base balance	700 mg	700 mg	Dairy, meat, poultry, fish, grains	Interfere with blood calcium levels
Magnesium	Energy production, metabolism of glucose, fats, and protein; important for bone health	400–420 mg	310–320 mg	Whole grains, leafy greens	Nausea, vomiting, low blood pressure, heart and kidney problems
Calcium	Bone and tooth formation; aids in nerve transmissions, blood clotting, and muscle contractions	1,000 mg	1,000 mg	Dairy products, tofu, kale, broccoli; fortified juice	Kidney stones and kidney disease
Iron	Prevents anemia; helps deliver oxygen to muscles	8 mg	18 mg	Meat, poultry, seafood, fortified cereals and grains	Gastrointestinal distress
Zinc	Essential for energy metabolism; aids in protein synthesis, immune system function, wound healing, and taste	11 mg	8 mg	Fortified cereals and grains; red meat, some seafood	Decreases copper
Selenium	Antioxidant, regulates thyroid hormone and enhances vitamin C status	55 mcg	55 mcg	Brazil nuts; oysters and clams; pork; pasta; poultry; sunflower seeds; meats; breads and oatmeal; soy; nuts; eggs	Loss of hair and brittle nails
Chromium	Helps control blood sugar levels	35 mcg	25 mcg	Meat, poultry, fish, some cereals, beer	Kidney problems

Vitamins D and K, pantothenic acid, biotin, and choline are Adequate Intakes.
*Based on adults 19–50 years old; not for pregnant or lactating women.

What's My EAR, DRI, or DV?

These may sound like some strange baseball stats, but they are technical terms issued by the Institute of Medicine (IOM) that tell us how much of a vitamin or a mineral we need each day. These form the basis of what are on food packages and supplement labels.

In the past, we had one set of guidelines, called the RDAs or recommended dietary allowances, but now the IOM has developed new terminology under the dietary reference intakes (DRIs). The DRIs contain four sets of values: (1) EARs, (2) RDAs, (3) AIs, and (4) ULs.

Here's what all the jargon stands for and what you need to know:

- **Estimated average requirement (EAR)** is a daily nutrient intake value that is estimated to meet the requirements of half of healthy individuals in specific age and gender groups.
- **Recommended dietary allowance (RDA)** is the gold standard for nutrient recommendations and is the average daily dietary intake sufficient to meet the nutrient requirements of virtually all (97 to 98 percent) healthy individuals in specific age and gender groups.
- **Adequate intake (AI)** is generally set for more emerging nutrients (such as choline and biotin) as an assumed nutritional goal when there is not enough scientific evidence to calculate an RDA.
- **Tolerable upper intake level (UL)** is the highest daily nutrient intake likely to pose no risk of adverse health effects for almost all individuals. Intakes above the UL may increase the risk of an adverse effect.
- **Daily value (DV)** is used on food labeling and supplement labels wherever there is a nutrition facts panel. It is the average amount of the vitamin or mineral needed to meet the nutritional requirements of a person of at least age four. The number shown will be the percentage of the daily value provided by one serving of the supplement.

Trusting What You Buy

If you choose to take a daily multivitamin and mineral supplement, do your homework first, as there are numerous cases of supplements that do not contain what is listed on the ingredients list, and some even have high levels of contaminants such as lead.

A good rule of thumb when purchasing vitamin and mineral supplements is to look for the USP (U.S. Pharmacopeia) Verified Dietary Supplement or the NSF International (The Public Health and Safety Company) dietary supplement certifications on the label. These are nonprofit organizations that test all types of dietary supplements to ensure that they are safe and deliver what they're supposed to. If a product bears either of these logos, you can be assured that it:

- delivers what is declared on the label;
- does not contain contaminants;
- is absorbable by the body;
- is manufactured using high-quality and purity standards.

10

The Athlete's Kitchen:
An Insider's Guide to the
Gold-Medal Eats

As sports dietitians, we have the chance to interact with thousands of athletes each year. Whether it's at events, online, or via one-on-one counseling, we have heard a lot of interesting sports nutrition tidbits from athletes from all walks of life. Following are real-life examples of world champions, Olympic gold medalists, and age groupers trying to find the energy so they can do what they have to do (read: work) with what they want to do (read: train). That's where we can really relate, as workaholics who also like to train and compete.

While we can provide you with all the calculations and science of how to eat a high-octane, performance-based diet, athletes have all the tricks of the trade for how to implement those guidelines into practice. They also let us know what's realistic given the unique circumstances athletes have to deal with concerning their diet and overall nutrition.

In the following material, we've outlined some of their best and worst practices, diet disasters, fave foods, superstitions, caffeine addictions, and tips for everything from making Nutella quesadillas and chocolate (gel) sundaes to PowerBar TripleThreat "recovery" milkshakes. To make you feel better, we'll tell you who loves In-N-Out burgers and nachos smothered in cheese.

Sports Nutrition Moment of Truth

We asked athletes to tell us about that moment when the skies parted, God spoke to them, or just when they bonked badly and suddenly realized nutrition could make or break their performance.

"While at UCLA, I took Physiological Science 5, better known as Diet and Exercise. We were required to record food intake and energy expenditures. I noticed that my food intake was very high, and that the all-you-can-eat accommodations in the on-campus dining halls were not the best thing for me. After talking with the instructor for the course, we decided it was important to strategize my food intake. My professor told me that my running achievements to date were the result of my genetics, despite my poor diet. Some of the steps I took to control eating were to eat some meals outside the dining halls, and to drink water before some meals, to lessen my appetite. This helped me achieve four NCAA championships the following year."

    —*Mebrahtom "Meb" Keflezighi, professional distance runner, U.S. Olympic medalist, marathon*

"I was on a really long, hard brick [bike-to-run] session and was about halfway through the run intervals. My legs were shattered and I thought I was going to have to call it a day. Then I took a packet of PowerBar Gel that had caffeine and I could run strong for the rest of the workout. It made me realize how just that little bit of carbohydrate could help salvage my workout."

    —*Samantha McGlone, professional triathlete, second-place finisher, 2007 Ironman World Championship*

"I lost ten pounds during the off-season, got stronger, and started winning races the next season."

    —*Peter Reid, three-time Ironman world champion*

"At the Ironman World Championship in 2000, I was running in the lead with Peter Reid. I started to fade a bit, but my legs were still feeling great. I couldn't quite figure out what was going on. When you begin to bonk, you don't think very clearly. As I approached a big hill, I saw a friend on the side of the road and said I didn't have any more energy. He yelled at me to EAT EVERYTHING! From there on I stuffed everything I could get my hands on in my mouth for several miles. My body responded, and I fought for the win, only to finish second. That stayed with me forever. It is pretty easy for me to recognize the effects of lacking calories now."

—*Tim DeBoom, two-time Ironman world champion*

"I competed in St. Anthony's triathlon in 1999 and I bonked with a mile to the finish and fell to the ground when I crossed the line. I had to be carried to the massage tent thinking I was just cramped up, but they insisted I get an IV instead. I did not want the IV, but they again insisted. Two IVs later, I got up and walked away as if I was fine all along. That's when I realized how quickly you can become dehydrated. Never again would I want to do that to myself, so I check my watch every fifteen minutes to be sure I am drinking on some sort of schedule."

—*Hollie Kenney, professional triathlete*

"I was running the Long Beach Marathon and it was 80+ degrees. I 'hit the wall,' largely due to dehydration, and I lost ten minutes over the last six miles and wound up on a saline drip for thirty minutes at the finish line. It's just not possible to get enough fluid by grabbing a half-filled cup of water at each five-mile aid station. In future events, I adapted by having my wife meet me several times out on the course with full water bottles and gels."

—*Kieran Sherlock, PowerBar Team elite member*

Diet Principles to Live By

In years past, we would meet athletes who were up to trying just about anything. They'd essentially eat tree bark if you told them it would boost their performance. And many were sustaining themselves on sports nutrition products, hardly the making for a well-balanced diet.

In the past five to ten years, we've seen athletes moving away from engineered foods and diets that relied heavily on a slew of supplements to having more healthful diets based on "real" foods and more wholesome ingredients. There is almost a movement among some away from any processed or unnatural products. (A trend coming not just from athletes in Boulder and Berkeley!)

The resounding diet that athletes are following is high in carbohydrates and lower in fats and proteins. Of course, one man's low-fat diet is another's high-fat, but the days of finding athletes trying to follow low- or moderate-carbohydrate diets such as the forty-thirty-thirty style of eating are few and far between.

Athletes also have gotten a better perspective about nutrition, allowing themselves to splurge when they feel like it. Others have found that they periodize their diet around their training, so that the volume and types of food they eat at one time of the year are completely different from what they eat during the season. Here are some of the overall diet philosophies provided to us:

"I periodize my nutrition based on my training. I eat lots of fruits and vegetables, lean protein (including red meat two to three times per week for the iron, since I live at altitude), and whole grains. I eat three to four meals/snacks per day based around my training schedule. Often this means a light snack in the morning before swim, a larger breakfast at around ten, then a snack pre- or post-training in the afternoon and then an early dinner. I eat most of my carbs early in the day to fuel training and then get in my higher-fiber and protein food (veggies and meats) at dinner. I add more carbs to dinner when I have a very long or hard workout the next morning."

—*Samantha McGlone, second place, 2007 Ironman World Championship*

"I balance my nutrition over a few days, so that I may not worry about one bad day of eating as long as the majority of the days are good."

—*Michael Johnson, nine-time world champion, Olympic gold medalist, sprinter*

"I am a very big believer in a balanced diet, with carbs, protein, and some good fat at all meals. I make sure there is a good source of protein with all meals so it's not just all carbs, and I eat four meals a day with a couple of snacks."

—*Peter Reid, three-time Ironman world champion*

"I periodize my meals and eat higher carbohydrates and less protein and fat before and after my workouts with more moderate amounts of carbs and more protein at all other times of the day."

—*Cody Wilson, BMX professional*

"Like all full-time working adults, it's tough to train, compete, and fit everything into one day. One thing that has really helped me is to eat nutritious foods. My definition of 'healthy' is whole grains, fruit and vegetables, and plenty of water. I avoid eating out as much as possible and I try to limit processed foods."

—*Samuel Wilson, triathlete and road cyclist*

"I try to eat home-cooked, organic, whole foods for my meals and snacks whenever I can. During hard training blocks and when racing, I increase carbohydrate and protein in my diet. I tend to eat several times throughout the day, with a big focus on breakfast."

—*Meredith Miller, professional cyclist*

The Athlete's Kitchen

We love the inside scoop about what athletes really eat when they're at home. Who has a fridge packed with Shiner Boch, and who has cupboards chockablock with candy and chocolate? Here's a look at some foods that athletes just cannot live without. You may be surprised at how "normally" these athletes eat, and most will be happy to hear that beer is still at the top of many athletes' must-have list.

Samantha McGlone, Professional Triathlete

Refrigerator	Pantry
Apples	Sweet chili sauce
Salad greens	Sea salt
Manna bread	Olive oil
Almond milk	Almond butter
Maple syrup	Red wine

Cody Wilson, Professional BMX Racer

Refrigerator	Pantry
Soy milk	Wheat tortilla/wraps
Egg substitute	High-fiber crackers
Chicken	High-fiber cereal
Turkey	Canned fruit
Yogurt	Canned veggies

Meredith Miller, Professional Cyclist

Refrigerator	Pantry
Silk soy milk	Newman's Own pretzels
Orange juice	Peanut butter
Fruit	Cereal
Cheese	Bread
Veggies	Dried fruit

Stuart Sheldon, Dynamo Water Polo Club, PowerBar Team Elite Member

Refrigerator	Pantry
Fresh fruit	PowerBar products
Cream cheese	Dried fruit
Broccoli	Nuts
Coke Zero	Canned soup
Shiner Boch	Beans

Josh Cox, Professional Distance Runner

Refrigerator	Pantry
Avocados	Rice
Water	Pasta
Corn tortillas	PowerBar products
Soy milk	Canned albacore tuna
Salad greens	Tea

Ruben Figueres, Elite Amateur Triathlete, PowerBar Team Elite Member

Refrigerator	Pantry
Milk	Recovery drink
Water	PowerBar Endurance
Bananas	Peanuts
Kiwis	Condensed milk
Cheese	PowerBar Nut Naturals

Michael Douglas, USAC Cycling Coach, Amateur Triathlete, and PowerBar Team Elite Member

Refrigerator	Pantry
Soy milk	PowerBar products
Apples	Cereal
Broccoli	Pasta
Diet Mountain Dew	Canned tomatoes
Beer	Whole-wheat pancake mix

Peter Reid, Three-time Ironman World Champion

Refrigerator	Pantry
Yogurt	Cereal (love muesli)
Apples	Rice
Veggies	Quinoa
Eggs	PowerBar products
Poultry or beef	Carbo Pro

Mebrahtom "Meb" Keflezighi, Professional Distance Runner, Olympian

Refrigerator	Pantry
Milk	Bagels
Orange juice	PowerBar products
Cottage cheese	Honey
Jelly	Supplements
Cream cheese	Bread

Energy to Burn Nutritionism: The top banana of fruit, is, well, bananas. Bananas are considered the perfect fruit because they are an excellent source of potassium, with more than four hundred milligrams per medium piece of fruit. Potassium is an electrolyte that is lost in small amounts in sweat, but it is not generally a cramp culprit, as many believe. Bananas also contain stomach-friendly carbs, are blendable for a great smoothie base, and come in a handy, naturally biodegradable package for on-the-go eating. A medium banana has the carbohydrates of a PowerBar Gel, twenty-five grams of carbs, and about a hundred calories. Bananas also have three grams of fiber, vitamin C, and B vitamins.

Preevent Pointers

Athletes' preevent choices run the gamut from Arby's to hippie cereals and Kozy Shack rice pudding. One thing that we hear from most elite-level athletes is that the more flexible you can be on your food choices, the better. This is because if you travel to events, you can never control what or when you can eat. Pros tell us that you need to be realistic about what you want versus what you can have. Your perfect or preferred meal may not be available, and you need to learn to make do with what is.

One thing most of the athletes can't do without, however, is their coffee or preevent caffeine fix. Our informal surveys suggest that coffee is much more popular than tea among athletes. We have athletes tell us all the time that they'd rather go without food than be deprived of their caffeine habit.

The Top Ten Preevent Favorites
- Coffee
- Oatmeal
- Ready-to-eat cereals
- Bagels with cream cheese and jam
- Pancakes or waffles
- Eggs and toast
- Fruit smoothies
- Pasta
- PowerBar products
- Peanut butter and jelly sandwiches

"Before the 2007 IronMan world championship I ate two pieces of wheat toast with almond butter, honey, and one banana; twenty ounces of Naked Juice; one cup of black coffee, about a thousand calories."

—Michael Lovato, *professional triathlete*

"I've learned that when racing in France, it's B.Y.O.B. or you may not make it to the finish line. As soon as I get to France, I buy cereal and other food in the supermarket and bring it to my hotel for my breakfasts."

—Kristin Armstrong, *2008 Olympic Gold Medalist, road cycling time trial*

"If it is an early game, then I will have eggs, pancakes, or cereal to get me off right, and I will bring a peanut butter and honey with me on the bus for something about 1½ hours before the game."

—*Brandi Chastain, Olympic soccer player*

"I will always start my day with a big bowl of cereal that usually consists of two to four types of cereal, fresh fruit, vanilla yogurt, and vanilla silk soymilk. "

—*Meredith Miller, professional cyclist*

"Eggs, toast, a 'hippie' cereal (like Kashi, Optimum), and coffee with Half & Half."

—*Jeff Louder, professional cyclist*

"If my race is before noon then I like to eat a big bowl of oatmeal with raisin and almonds on top. If my race begins in the early or late afternoon I will have oatmeal with raisins and almonds as well as a peanut butter and jelly about an hour and a half before I start (two hours before a TT)."

—*Kristin Armstrong, professional cyclist*

"Before the 2007 Hawaii Ironman world championship I ate two packets of organic instant oatmeal and a triple espresso. I abstain from coffee the week before a big event (I can only do this once a year!) and then have a triple espresso on race morning for an extra kick."

—*Samantha McGlone, professional triathlete*

"Coffee, half a bagel, coffee, half a Cappuccino PowerBar Performance Bar, coffee, the second half of my bagel, coffee, the second half of the performance bar, coffee, coffee, and some more coffee, then a gel just before the start."

—*Josh Cox, professional distance runner*

"I try not to get too dependent on any specific foods, prerace or otherwise. You will always run into a situation when things don't go right, and you don't get what you are used to. You have to be able to adapt. I like to call it developing a steel gut. I used to not be able to stomach much because of nerves, so I stuck with liquids and possibly some bland toast. Recently, I've switched to French toast as my prerace meal. I think I just needed to find something that I truly loved and could always stomach in any situation."

—*Tim DeBoom, two-time Ironman world champion*

What makes oatmeal the most popular preevent food? Oats are a whole grain that pack in about 120 to 160 calories per one-cup cooked serving (half a cup raw), depending upon the brand and if it's flavored. A cup of oatmeal packs in four to five grams of protein and three to four grams of fiber, and part of that fiber is the cholesterol-cutting soluble fiber beta-glucan. More than forty studies have proven that oatmeal helps lower cholesterol, and other studies show that it helps with weight management, blood pressure, and type 2 diabetes. And whether you eat instant, quick-cooking, or steel-cut, all oatmeals are made from the same oat groat, are whole grains, and confer the same health benefits. From a performance perspective, protein may provide the perfect combination of protein and fiber to keep you fuller longer but not too much fiber to cause GI distress. Rice cookers make steel-cut oats perfect every time. Set your rice cooker on a timer, put your oats, water, and raisins in at bedtime, and voilà! breakfast will be ready even before your coffee.

Favorite Food Indulgences

Even the most disciplined of athletes give in to their favorite food cravings. They just do it in moderation or they burn so many calories with training that they can afford more sugar, fat-rich treats, or alcohol.

"Viva la guacamole!!! As often as possible! Instead of eating guac with fried chips, I buy corn tortillas, cut them into quarters, and heat them in the oven for fresh, hot-baked tortilla chips."
—Josh Cox, *professional distance runner*

"In-N-Out burgers and fries. I want it every time I drive from Mammoth to San Diego."
—Mebrahtom "Meb" Keflezighi, *professional distance runner, U.S. Olympic medalist, marathon*

"Wine is probably my biggest weakness, though. I have wine a few times a week during the week and definitely on the weekend."
—Michael Johnson, *Olympic track sprinter*

"Beer and nachos on Saturday night with my local buddies at the pub. I call it cheat night. I am allowed one of those a week so that I am somewhat strict the rest of the week."
—Peter Reid, *three-time Ironman world champion*

"Diet Coke . . . I drink it daily. I drink about three cans a day."
—*Kristin Armstrong, 2008 Olympic Gold Medalist, road cycling time trial*

"ICE CREAM!!! No more than twice per week."
—*Tom Romano, PowerBar Team elite member*

"Sweets! Candy, baked goods, but I try to keep it to once a month."
—*Cody Wilson, pro BMXer*

"I love pizza or Chinese food and ice cream. I limit myself to once a month and out of season."
—*Kevin Matthews, Cat I track rider and PowerBar Team elite member*

"I love chocolate and eat some almost every day. I try to stick to dark, but I also have a weakness for peanut M&Ms."
—*Samantha McGlone, professional triathlete*

"I definitely have a sweet tooth, and the rule of thumb that I try to follow is if I have sweets, to have 'quality' ones, like Ben & Jerry's ice cream. I also enjoy a glass of wine about four times a week. In terms of my sweet tooth, I allow myself something small once a day."
—*Kathryn Curi Mattis, professional cyclist*

"Chocolate chip pancakes. I eat them once a month or so. I usually don't feel too good afterward, though."
—*Hollie Kenney, professional triathlete*

Diet Disasters

One of the best ways to learn how to do things is to fail first or just learn from those who have experienced a full-on sports nutrition meltdown. Here, some horror stories:

"Before a game against Japan, one of my teammates who was (is) battling Epstein-Barr syndrome was in a juicing trend. I love veggies and fruits, so I told her I would have one. Well, thirty-two ounces of delicious juice later, I had the worst stomach cramps and we had about an hour before our warm-up. I couldn't get off the floor and could barely move for the entire warm-up. I returned to the locker room, where finally I was able to rid myself of the gas (thanks to some more curling up and some Tums). That was the worst pain I had experienced due to food or drink."

—*Brandi Chastain, U.S. Women's Soccer Team, Olympic gold medalist*

"I did an Ironman in Nice, France, and all was going great on the bike. I was feeling strong and my nutrition had been really smooth. Then I missed my special-needs bag at the halfway point and didn't get any calories for the last eighty kilometers of the bike. That didn't put me in a good situation for the run. The wheels fell off. There was no way I could make up the calories I missed, and I did quite a bit of walking to finish the race and saw my hopes of winning go out the window. This made me always have two or three backup plans for every situation that could happen."

—*Tim DeBoom, two-time Hawaii Ironman world champion*

"I was in Japan at a World Cup and ate sushi for lunch the day before the race. My stomach was a little upset that evening so I chewed a Pepto-Bismol tablet and went to bed. On race morning I woke up and my tongue was entirely black. I was really worried that I was seriously ill and considered going to the hospital instead of the race start. I ended up having one of my best races ever and it turns out that black tongue is actually a side effect of the Pepto. . . . Who knew?"

—*Samantha McGlone, professional triathlete*

The Top Ten Most-Feared Foods

These are the foods athletes told us they try to avoid due to their poor nutritional quality, high saturated fat content, or, in some cases, the vegetarian lifestyle that many athletes follow.

1. Fast food
2. Fried food
3. Sugar substitutes
4. Hydrogenated oils
5. Soda
6. Candy
7. Baked goods
8. Overly processed packaged products
9. Red meat (vegetarian athletes)
10. Dairy (vegetarian athletes)

Train Your Sports Nutrition: Tips from the Top

PowerBar's professional and top amateur athletes often have great tricks to keep hydrated and carbohydrate stores stocked during exercise. Here are some of their best tips:

"Don't keep it in the house; then it's easier not to eat. At work, I structure my schedule and workday to not be near lunch spreads near meeting rooms, and eat yogurt and drink calorie-free drinks like tea upon arriving; that seems to reduce the hunger cycles later in the day. If I come in and get working on an empty stomach, then I'll end up with appetite whiplash later in the day."

"At work I had a Post-it on my computer that said, 'Remember Your Goals.' I just think how hard I have worked on the bike to put in the training and my body deserves to be fed high-quality food."

"The hardest thing to do is to balance good nutrition with travel. Stay away from restaurants and close to health food stores."

"Proper nutrition takes planning. Make sure you have bottles of sports drinks that you can access during your training. Always bring fruit and a protein bar to eat postworkout. Proper recovery and proper nutrition begin the moment the workout ends."

"Always drink when others are drinking around you."

"Use sports nutrition products; they work."

"A lot of people exercise on an empty stomach, but eating a small snack before doing any physical activity will improve the workout."

"Learn to be more flexible about your diet. This will help when competing when things won't always go your way and you may not get your preferred outcome."

"Travel with foods you love to help ensure that you have your faves with you."

"When traveling for competitions, stay somewhere with a kitchen so you can prepare your own meals. Rent a condo, choose a hotel with kitchenettes, or arrange for a home stay through the race organization."

The Top Ten Kitchen Utensil Must-Haves

It may be that sports and nutrition are so entwined, or that food is often a reward for a hard workout, but athletes' culinary skills always amaze us.

While we haven't met many athletes who double as chefs, we are sure there are some. Most have a standard repertoire of dishes that they can whip up at a moment's notice, and they will talk All-Clad versus cast-iron skillets and the right set of knives that get the job done.

The must-haves that athletes tell us that they cannot live without in their kitchens:

1. Blender
2. Coffee maker
3. Microwave
4. Colander
5. Steamer
6. Great knives
7. Rice cooker
8. Salad spinner
9. Cast-iron skillet
10. Large pot for pasta

Recipes from Professional Athletes

Kelly White, M.S., R.D., C.S.S.D.
Board-Certified Sports Dietitian and Ironman Competitor

WHOLE-GRAIN APPLE BLUEBERRY BAKE

Serve for dessert, or when cooled, add yogurt or milk and have it for breakfast!

3 medium-size apples
1½ cups fresh blueberries

Crust:
½ cup whole wheat flour
½ cup rolled oats
½ cup unsweetened applesauce
¼ tsp cinnamon
2½ tbsp canola oil

Dice apples with skin on and pour into pie dish (does not need to be sprayed). Pour blueberries on top of apples.

Mix crust until thoroughly mixed and thick. Spread crust evenly over fruit mixture.

Bake in oven at 375–400 degrees.

Pamela M. Nisevich, M.S., R.D., L.D.

Consultant Sports and Wellness Dietitian, Nutrition for the Long Run Marathoner

POWER ON OATMEAL

½ cup old-fashioned rolled oats, dry
½ cup skim milk or low-fat soy milk
½ cup water
¼ cup chopped, dried mixed fruit (including prunes, apricots, and pears)
¼ cup chopped black walnuts

Combine oats, skim milk (soy milk, if using), and water.

Heat in microwave for about 45 seconds or until mixture begins to boil.

Stir. Add dried fruit and nuts.

Return to microwave for approximately 15–20 seconds, or until mixture returns to a boil.

Allow oatmeal to cool before serving.

Tricia L. Griffin, R.D., C.S.S.D.

Sports Nutritionist, Performance Nutrition

BREAKFAST BURRITO

Great for a pregame light meal on the go!

Makes 2

3 ounces skim milk
2–3 large eggs
Onion and garlic powder to taste
Pinch basil
4 ounces low-fat shredded cheddar cheese
2 large flour tortillas
1–2 tbsp mild salsa; optional

Mix milk, eggs, and spices in a bowl. Cook over low heat, add cheese. Cook until eggs are solid. Place in tortilla, add salsa. Roll up and enjoy!

Tom Morton

*PGA Director of Player Development for Morton Gold
in Sacramento, California*

BLUE CHEESE TURKEY BURGERS

2 servings

1 sweet yellow onion	2 hamburger buns
½ lb turkey burger	1 tsp olive oil
1 tbsp Worcestershire	1 tsp sugar
Garlic salt and pepper	1 tbsp balsamic vinegar
2 oz blue cheese (2 small cubes)	Grey Poupon mustard

Slice onion into thin strips. Set aside.

Season turkey burger meat with 1 tbsp Worcestershire, pepper, and garlic salt. Form into round balls. Stuff each burger with a cube of blue cheese, flatten into thick patty, making sure cheese is not exposed. Grill on barbecue for 15 minutes or until done. Put buns on grill last couple of minutes to warm.

Once you put the burgers on the grill, sauté onions in pan with olive oil on medium heat for 5 minutes, stirring occasionally. After 5 minutes, adjust to low heat and add sugar and balsamic vinegar. Cook for another 15 minutes on low, stirring occasionally. Onions will carmelize.

Add Grey Poupon to bun and top burger with carmelized onions. Enjoy!

Danna Brown

Road and Mountain Biking

CHOCOLATE PUDDING

¼ cup flour	¼ cup dark cocoa powder or dark
⅓ cup water	chocolate pieces
⅔ cup sugar	1½ cups skim milk
2 egg yolks	1 tbsp vanilla

In a large saucepan, stir together first five ingredients, making sure there are no lumps. Add milk and cook over medium heat until thickened. Stir occasionally at first, then constantly after it begins steaming, remove from heat when you see the first bubble (do not boil). Add vanilla immediately, then stop stirring. Cover with Saran Wrap to avoid "skin."

EGGPLANT FUSION

Serves 4 generously as appetizer

1 large eggplant
1 tbsp miso paste
2 tbsp orange juice
2 tsp sugar
5 plum tomatoes, coarsely chopped

¾ cup loosely packed baby arugula
  or chopped arugula
1 tbsp extra virgin olive oil (or
  orange-infused olive oil)
4 whole-wheat pitas

Pierce eggplant several times with fork. Roast at 400 degrees about 30 min. Meanwhile, whisk together miso, orange juice, and sugar, and allow to dissolve. When eggplant is cool enough to work with, remove skin and chop coarsely. Combine in serving bowl with tomato and miso mixture. Gently toss in arugula. Drizzle with olive oil.

Cut pita into wedges, lightly toast in 400-degree oven, and serve with eggplant dip.

Leigh Crews
Yoga/Pilates

SWEET POTATO AND BLACK BEAN
STUFFED CHILIES

1 large sweet potato or 1 can yams,
  rinsed and drained
7 oz or ½ can black beans
7 oz of your favorite salsa

1 can mild green chilies, whole,
  roasted, and peeled
3–4 oz reduced-fat Mexican cheese

Microwave or boil the sweet potato until tender. Mash with the black beans. Add salsa and season to taste. Fill the chili peppers with the sweet potato mixture. Sprinkle with reduced-fat shredded Mexican cheese. Bake in 350-degree oven for 30 minutes or until heated through, or microwave until hot. Serve with brown rice and a salad. *Note:* The sweet potato mixture is also delicious in a wrap with sliced deli chicken and shredded cabbage.

Amy Hutchison

Cycling and Triathlon, Team Bi-Lo

LIVE BROWNIES

3 cups walnuts	¼ cup raw carob
1 cup sunflower seeds	2 tbsp coconut oil
4 dry dates (pitted)	Pinch of sea salt
4 soaked dates (pitted)	1 tsp vanilla extract
½ cup shredded coconut	¼ cup agave nectar

Grind walnuts in food processor until fine, then place in bowl. Grind sunflower seeds in food processor until fine. Add dry dates to the sunflower seeds in the processor while it is on, then add soaked dates while the processor is on until a large ball forms. Add coconut oil, carob, and sea salt to walnuts and mix. Next add vanilla and agave to the walnut mixture. Combine the dough ball with the walnut mixture. Press into a 9" loaf pan and garnish with coarsely chopped walnuts. Cut into squares or bars.

Suzanne Stonebarger

AVP Pro Beach Volleyball Player

BAKED HALIBUT WITH BRUSCHETTA

Preheat oven to 375 degrees. Cook fillets on a foil-lined cookie sheet for 15–18 minutes. Squeeze lemon and a splash of olive oil onto the fillets.

Add a scoop of bruschetta (recipe below) to each fillet with 5 minutes remaining:

Bruschetta	
1–2 tbsp chopped garlic	½ cup olive oil
1 tbsp olive oil	¼ cup balsamic vinegar
4 to 5 Roma tomatoes	Salt and pepper to taste
1 bunch fresh basil	1 baguette

Sauté garlic with olive oil on medium heat. Dice tomatoes and place in bowl. Chop fresh basil leaves or process lightly in food processor. Add ¼ cup olive oil, balsamic vinegar, and blend with cooked garlic. Add salt and pepper to taste.

Preheat oven to 450 degrees. Slice the baguette diagonally into ½-inch-thick slices. Spread one side of each slice with remaining olive oil.

Place on cookie sheet with olive oil side down on top rack of oven. Brown the slices for 5–6 minutes. Take the slices out of the oven and top with the tomato-basil mixture with olive oil side up.

Steve Ilg

Nordic Skiing, Ski Racing, Quadrathlon, Snowshoe Racing, Running, Yoga

MUSCLE-UP MANICOTTI

*Trust me: the prep time is a great passive meditation before
a race or hard workout day, and your patience will be well
rewarded by soaring levels of muscle glycogen!*

Preparation time: 50 minutes
Serves: 3–4

8 oz soy or regular low-fat
mozzarella
¾ cube hard tofu, crumbled
1 bunch spinach, steamed and
cooled
½ onion, steamed along with
spinach

28 oz tomato sauce
8 oz manicotti, precooked and
cooled
Optional: ½–¾ cups Parmesan,
grated

Preheat oven to 350 degrees. In a mixing bowl combine cheese, tofu, spinach, and onion (filling). Prepare a lasagna pan by pouring ¼" tomato sauce over bottom. Carefully fill each manicotti by hand. Place each filled manicotti into lasagna pan. Do not stack the manicotti. When done, pour the rest of the tomato sauce over the pasta. Cover the top lightly with foil and bake for 25 minutes. Uncover and spread grated Parmesan on top (this step is optional). Bake for another 5 minutes. Serve.

Steve and Wendy Panetta

Tennis

PROTEIN BARS

2 cups or 1 16-oz jar natural peanut
butter
1–1¾ cups honey*

2¼ cups whey chocolate or vanilla
protein powder
3 cups dry uncooked oats

Combine peanut butter and honey in a microwave-safe bowl. Heat for about 60 seconds or until peanut butter is creamy and stirs easily. Add protein powder and regular or quick-cooking oats. (Do not use steel-cut oats.) Blend all ingredients. Press into a 9"-by-16" pan. Refrigerate for 1 hour or until solid enough to cut into bars. Wrap each bar in foil or plastic wrap.

*After much experimentation with the recipe, I have found that one 12-oz jar of honey keeps these bars yummy and reduces the sugar content by almost half; 12 ounces of honey = 1 cup. Each bar would have about 300 calories with reduced honey.

Diane Proud
Triathlete

GREEN EGGS IN A PAN

Olive oil cooking spray

2 organic eggs (or omega 3–enriched eggs)

2–3 cups organic mixed salad greens and/or spinach

Salt and pepper to taste

Optional: tortilla, English muffin, salsa, grated cheese, or condiments of choice

Utensils:

small sauté pan or frying pan with lid

spatula

Turn burner to medium-high heat. Spray small pan with olive oil cooking spray.

Crack open 2 eggs in pan, sunny side up. Immediately cover eggs with greens and place lid on pan.

The greens wilt from steam created in the pan. After a minute or so, turn burner off, allowing eggs to finish cooking to preferred doneness as burner heat subsides.

Serve alone or on top of a whole-grain tortilla or English muffin.

Jamie Tidmore
Kayak

FAST AND EASY BEANS AND RICE

This is a healthy, simple recipe for athletes on the go when you are just too tired after a long day training to put a lot of time into dinner but want something yummy and nutritious.

1 small package frozen spinach

1 small package frozen corn kernels

1 can black beans

1–2 tsp chili powder

1 tsp garlic powder

1 medium onion

1 tbsp olive oil

2 cups cooked white or brown rice

½ cup shredded low-fat cheese

Hot sauce or salsa verde to taste

Thaw spinach and corn in microwave. Drain excess water.

In separate bowl drain beans and spice them up with the chili and garlic powder.

In large sauté pan, cook onion with olive oil. Add beans, spinach, and corn. Stir and cook until all ingredients soften.

Mix beans, spinach, and corn with the onion. Stir to cover everything with chili powder and cook to warm.

Serve over rice and top with cheese, hot sauce, or salsa verde.

Sharon Beltrandelrio
Triathlete

DELICIOUS HEALTHY CHEESECAKE

Crust
1 cup whole-wheat flour
1 cup oats
2 tablespoons sugar

¼ cup milk
¼ cup olive oil

Combine all ingredients. Form into a pie crust using a rolling pin. Place on bottom of greased 9" pie pan. (Can substitute a store-bought pie crust, but it's probably not as healthy.)

Cheesecake
8 oz reduced-fat cream cheese
1 cup nonfat plain yogurt
14 oz nonfat sweetened condensed milk

2 eggs
½ cup fresh-squeezed lime juice
1 teaspoon vanilla

Combine all ingredients. Blend until smooth. Pour into prepared pie crust. Bake at 350 degrees for 50 minutes or until center is set.

Amanda Durner
Triathlete

TAMARI ALMONDS

1 package raw almonds
(14 oz)

½ cup tamari sauce (Asian aisle in grocery)

Place almonds in glass pie dish and cook in microwave for 2½ minutes on high; take out and stir.

Pour tamari sauce over almonds, enough to cover almonds. Stir so tamari and almonds are mixed and covered . . . a little tamari on bottom of dish is okay!

Put back in microwave for 2½ minutes on high, remove, and place almonds on cookie sheet to cool.

CITRUS-ROSEMARY SALMON

4 large salmon fillets
Olive oil
Kosher salt or sea salt
Pepper, freshly ground

1 orange, 2 lemons, and 2 limes, plus slices of these fruits for garnish

Place salmon in Pyrex dish or baking pan.

Drizzle oil over both sides of fillets. Add salt and pepper and then squeeze the juice of the orange, lemons, and limes over the fillets. Lay the rosemary sprigs in the pan and over the fillets. Cover and place in refrigerator overnight for best results.

Grill or bake salmon fillets. Squeeze more orange/lemon/lime juice over fillets if needed. Once cooked, place fillets on a clean serving platter and garnish with orange, lemon, and lime circle slices and fresh rosemary sprigs.

Matt Pelletier

Runner

SWEET POTATO QUESADILLAS

Makes 4 large quesadillas

1 large sweet potato
8 medium-size wraps (tortilla-size)
Taco seasoning (to taste)

Salsa, hot sauce, and guacamole to taste

Preheat oven to 400 degrees.

Peel the sweet potato, and cut it into small blocks (the peels can be baked into sweet potato fries). Boil the sweet potato blocks until tender. Mash the sweet potato. Place 2 wraps on a baking sheet, cover each wrap with a thin layer of sweet potato dusted with taco seasoning (optional). Cover each filled wrap with a second wrap (creating a sandwich). Bake at 400 degrees for 10 minutes, or until outside of quesadilla becomes slightly browned and crispy. Top with salsa, hot sauce, guacamole, or even sour cream to taste.

This recipe was given to me by one of my vegetarian training partners and his wife. It's quick, easy to make, and very inexpensive.

AVOSALSA

Makes 24 small servings, but I tend to put it on everything, so it doesn't last long.

6 pitted, peeled, and diced avocados
3 large, diced tomatoes
½ cup finally chopped red onion
4 cloves minced garlic

6 tbsp chopped fresh cilantro
Juice of 1 large lime
1½ tsp ground cumin
¾ tsp sea salt
¾ tsp freshly ground pepper

In a large bowl, combine all ingredients. I use a food processor for the cilantro, onion, and garlic, as it saves a lot of time.

Make sure not to liquefy the avocados and tomatoes to maintain a chunky consistency.

This recipe was originally from an online recipe, but it has been modified to its state of perfection.

Aaron Kamnetz

Triathlete

SPICY GREEN BEANS WITH GARLIC AND GINGER

2 lb green beans	⅛–¼ tsp red pepper flakes
3 tbsp vegetable oil	½ tsp salt
2 garlic cloves, minced	2 tbsp soy sauce
1 tsp minced fresh ginger	

Boil beans until tender for about 10 minutes; drain and cool.

In wok or frying pan, heat oil over medium-high heat, add garlic, and cook until fragrant. Add ginger and pepper flakes and cook 15 seconds. Raise heat to high, add beans and salt, and cook, stirring constantly until heated through for 1–2 minutes. Add soy sauce and cook until soy sauce is reduced to a glaze. Serve.

Michael Wardian

Runner

BANANA BREAD

½ cup butter	1¼ cups flour
1 cup sugar	¾ tsp baking soda
2 eggs	½ tsp salt
¾ cup ripe mashed bananas (about 2)	

Preheat oven to 350 degrees.
Cream butter and sugar until fluffy.
Add eggs and beat well.
Stir in mashed bananas.
Sift in dry ingredients.
Mix well.
Bake for 30–35 minutes in an ungreased loaf pan.

Leanda Cave

Professional Triathlete

CHICKEN CURRY

Serves: 4–6 adults
Prep time: 30 minutes
Cook time: 30 minutes

2 chicken breasts chopped in strips
(turkey or tofu can be used as
substitutes)
1 tbsp peanut/sesame oil
A mix of vegetables; any of the
following or your favorites
1 red pepper chopped in strips
1 yellow pepper chopped in
strips
1 cup sugar snap peas cut in half
12 baby corns chopped in thirds
1 red/brown onion chopped in
strips

1–2 tbsp mild curry powder
(depending on taste)
1 tbsp crushed ginger
1 tbsp crushed garlic
3 tbsp honey
1 can coconut milk
½ cup water
3 tbsp soy sauce
16 oz Chinese wheat noodles
(or angel hair pasta cooked)
1 tbsp corn flour mixed with
¼ cup water

In large, nonstick fry pan or wok, fry meat/tofu until cooked. Add vegetables and cook until slightly tender. Add all the other ingredients except noodles and corn flour and bring to boil. Add noodles and simmer for 5 minutes or until noodles have cooked. Add corn flour and stir until thickened. Serve immediately.

Sarah Stiner

Runner

YOGURT BREAKFAST BLEND

This is a great meal to start off the day and full of flavor!

1 cup plain yogurt
1 banana sliced
½ cup strawberries sliced

2 tbsp raisins
¼ cup grape nuts
Honey to sweeten

Nick Weber

Surfer

THE POWER EGG SCRAMBLE

Onion
Roma tomato
Turkey sausage
2 cups spinach

3 egg whites
1 full egg
Parmesan cheese

Sauté onion, tomato, and turkey sausage. Add just-rinsed spinach to medley. Once the onions are clear and sausage is cooked, add mixed-up eggs and Parmesan cheese to medley, scramble or omelette style, whichever you prefer.

Megan Metcalfe

NCAA Champion, Middle-Distance Track

MEG'S MEATLOAF

2 cups bran flakes, mashed
1 cup barbecue sauce, divided
3 egg whites
1 lb bison meat
1 medium onion

½ cup shredded carrots
1 medium green pepper
½ cup mushrooms
1 can corn
2 tbsp garlic

Preheat oven to 375 degrees. Mix cereal, ½ cup barbecue sauce, and egg whites until blended. Add remaining ingredients and mix. Pat into baking dish. Brush with rest of barbecue sauce. Bake 1 hour, until meat is cooked through.

Enjoy! This recipe is iron-packed and is great as leftovers.

Kierann Smith

Runner and Second-Year Medical Student at Stanford

BROILED CHICKEN AND
RED PEPPERS ON A PITA

Time from start to finish: 20 minutes

4 servings

⅓ cup olive oil
¼ tsp dried oregano
½ tsp ground cumin
¾ tsp salt
½ tsp black pepper
1½ lb boneless chicken, cut into
    2½" cubes

1 red (or orange or yellow) bell
    pepper, cut lengthwise into
    ½"-wide strips
1 medium red onion, cut length-
    wise into ½" strips
Whole-wheat pita bread
8–10 oz prepared hummus (I like
    Tribe plain or roasted garlic)

Preheat the broiler and line a shallow baking pan with aluminum foil.

In a large bowl mix olive oil, oregano, cumin, salt, and pepper. Toss with chicken and vegetables. Spread into baking pan and broil 4–6 inches from heat for 8 minutes, stirring halfway through, until chicken is cooked and vegetables are slightly charred.

Toast the pita bread while the vegetables are in the oven (works great if you have a toaster oven; otherwise just throw them in the oven with the chicken and vegetables for the last 1–2 minutes), then spread the hummus on pitas, and finally top with chicken and vegetables.

So delicious, so easy, and not a lot of ingredients. I love pitas and hummus; I usually eat carrots and hummus while preparing if I am really hungry. I've also used zucchini and even asparagus in this recipe; lots of different vegetables can fit! The red onions are so delicious in this recipe, and they are cheap!

Tina Pic

Professional Road Cyclist
Colavita/Sutter Home Presented by Cooking Light

PASTA WITH PESTO AND SHRIMP

Cook shrimp in frying pan with a little olive oil, coriander, some red pepper, salt, pepper, and garlic.

Meanwhile, cook one box of angel hair pasta or linguine.

Pesto Sauce
2–3 cups fresh basil leaves, packed
½ cup freshly grated Parmesan-
   Reggiano or Romano cheese
½ cup pine nuts or walnuts

2–3 medium-size garlic cloves,
   minced
¾ cup extra virgin olive oil
Salt and freshly ground black
   pepper to taste

Process basil, cheese, nuts, and garlic in a food processor. Add olive oil slowly while processing ingredients.

Finish by adding salt and pepper to taste.

Top pasta with pesto and shrimp. Serve immediately.

11

The Fourteen-Day Energy
to Burn Diet

Now that you have the know-how to create a nutrition strategy for your active lifestyle, and suggestions from the elite, we think it's time to create a diet that works for you! To get you started, we have carefully created a fourteen-day meal plan for a 2,500-calorie diet. You can rest assured that these meals are nutrient-packed, generous in vitamins and minerals, meet your fiber needs, and give you the right ratios of carbohydrates, proteins, and good fats.

The Energy to Burn Diet plan includes:

- detailed recipes, instructions, and a shopping list
- complete nutrient analysis
- the right ratio of carbohydrates, proteins, and good fats:
  - 55–65 percent of total calories from carbohydrates; 25–35 g of fiber
  - 15–20 percent of total calories from proteins
  - 20–30 percent of total calories from fats; less than 10 percent from saturated fats, and trans fats as low as possible

We also understand the importance of a whole-grain-, fruits-, and vegetable-based diet with lean meats and nutritious recipes. We combined this with easy-to-follow, convenient choices that will give you energy and easily fit into your active lifestyle.

The Energy to Burn Diet: 2,500 Calories

Day 1
Breakfast
    1 cup of oatmeal made from ⅓ cup dry oats and ¾ cup nonfat milk

    1 tbsp natural peanut butter (mixed into oatmeal); you can substitute almond butter, walnut butter, or soy-nut butter for peanut butter

    1 medium banana

    10 oz nonfat milk

Lunch
    Quinoa salad (see recipe page 217)

    1 medium banana, sliced

    ½ cup low-fat cottage cheese

Dinner
    1 cup minestrone soup

    Chicken Caesar salad

        2 cups chopped romaine lettuce

        1 tbsp shredded Parmesan cheese

        2 tbsp fat-free Caesar dressing

        3 oz sliced, grilled chicken

    1 garlic-Parmesan bread stick

    1½ servings (about 12 oz) homemade lasagna (see recipe page 218)

    1 cup whole strawberries

Snacks
    1 medium Bartlett pear

    12 oz fruit smoothie

Nutrition	Total kilocalories: 2,516	Grams of carbohydrates: 365
Facts	Percent of calories from carbohydrates: 58	Grams of proteins: 129
	Percent of calories from proteins: 18	Grams of fats: 60
	Grams of saturated fats: 18.5 (7%)	Grams of trans fats: 0
	Percent of calories from fats: 22	Grams of fiber: 34

Day 2
Breakfast
2 slices 100% whole-wheat toast

1 tbsp reduced-fat spread

1 tbsp 100% fruit preserves

2 egg whites cooked in 1 tbsp reduced-fat spread

1 cup cantaloupe, cubed

6 oz nonfat, light (reduced-sugar) yogurt

Lunch
Macaroni and cheese (see recipe page 219)

1 cup diced pineapple

Dinner
Roasted vegetables with brown rice pasta (see recipe page 219)

Quick and easy salad (see recipe page 220)

½ cup low-fat cottage cheese

1 cup diced pineapple

Snacks
2 oz animal crackers

3 tbsp raisins

Nutrition *Facts*	Total kilocalories: 2,550	Grams of carbohydrates: 370
	Percent of calories from carbohydrates: 59	Grams of proteins: 119
	Percent of calories from proteins: 18	Grams of fats: 66
	Grams of saturated fats: 14.6 (5%)	Grams of trans fats: 0
	Percent of calories from fats: 23	Grams of fiber: 40

Day 3
Breakfast
1 cup wheat bran flakes cereal

8 oz nonfat milk

1 cup red grapes

1 large egg lightly fried in 1 tbsp reduced-fat spread

Lunch

Tomato and basil pizza (see recipe page 220)

Salad with walnut dressing (see recipe page 220)

6 oz nonfat (fruit on the bottom or blended) yogurt

½ cup blueberries

Dinner

1 cup hot and sour Chinese soup (ready to serve from a can or home-made)

1½ cups cooked wild rice, tossed with 1 tbsp sesame oil

7 oz steamed shrimp

1 cup steamed mixed vegetables

¾ cup citrus fruit sorbet

3 tbsp fat-free chocolate syrup

Snacks

1 toasted, 100% whole-wheat English muffin

2 tsp jam or preserves

Nutrition Facts	Total kilocalories: 2,476	Grams of carbohydrates: 341
	Percent of calories from carbohydrates: 55	Grams of proteins: 125
	Percent of calories from proteins: 20	Grams of fats: 68
	Grams of saturated fats: 15.6 (6%)	Grams of trans fats: 0
	Percent of calories from fats: 25	Grams of fiber: 30

Day 4

Breakfast

1 whole-wheat pita filled with

    2 egg whites cooked in 1 tbsp light spread

    1 slice low-fat American cheese

    2 slices tomato

1 large apple

8 oz milk

Lunch

1 cup cooked long-grain brown rice

6 oz grilled salmon basted with

2 tbsp brown sugar

1 tsp olive oil

8 asparagus spears

2 Parker House dinner rolls (from bakery)

1 cup fresh fruit, including citrus

Dinner

1 serving Mexican tortilla bake (see recipe page 221)

1 cup sliced cucumber

1 tbsp balsamic vinegar

1 tsp olive oil

¾ cup nonfat vanilla frozen yogurt

½ cup sliced strawberries

Snacks

2 fig cookies

8 oz 100% fruit juice

Nutrition	Total kilocalories: 2,497	Grams of carbohydrates: 332
Facts	Percent of calories from carbohydrates: 54	Grams of proteins: 128
	Percent of calories from proteins: 20	Grams of fats: 73
	Grams of saturated fats: 14 (5%)	Grams of trans fats: 0
	Percent of calories from fats: 26	Grams of fiber: 32

Day 5

Breakfast

Omelet consisting of

¼ cup chopped green bell pepper

¼ cup chopped red ripe tomato

¼ cup drained, canned mushrooms

2 large whole eggs

1 large egg white

1 slice low-fat cheddar cheese

1 tbsp reduced-fat spread

2 slices 100% whole-wheat toast

1 cup fruit cocktail canned in natural juices

Lunch

Nontraditional Caesar salad

    3 oz grilled chicken cooked with

        1 tbsp olive oil

    4 cups chopped romaine lettuce

    1 tbsp grated Parmesan cheese

    2 tbsp sun-dried tomatoes

    ¼ cup golden raisins

    Sprinkle balsamic vinegar to taste

1 toasted, whole-wheat pita

2 tbsp hummus

1 cup strawberry halves

Dinner

6 oz broiled pork tenderloin, lean

1 small baked sweet potato, topped with

    2 tbsp spread made with olive oil

    1 tsp ground cinnamon

    2 tbsp brown sugar, packed

1 cup cooked green beans

½ cup cranberry orange relish

Snacks

1 PowerBar Pria 110 Plus bar, any flavor

8 oz nonfat milk

Nutrition	Total kilocalories: 2,494	Grams of carbohydrates: 319
Facts	Percent of calories from carbohydrates: 51	Grams of proteins: 138
	Percent of calories from proteins: 22	Grams of fats: 75
	Grams of saturated fats: 17 (5.5%)	Grams of trans fats: 0
	Percent of calories from fats: 27	Grams of fiber: 34

Day 6

Breakfast

6 oz nonfat (fruit on the bottom or blended) yogurt

½ cup low-fat granola (without raisins)

2 large eggs cooked in 1 tbsp vegetable oil spread

2 pieces 100% whole-wheat toast

1 medium Bartlett pear

Lunch

Fajitas made with

   3 oz sautéed flank steak

   ¼ cup chopped green bell pepper

   ¼ cup chopped red bell pepper

   ¼ cup chopped yellow bell pepper

   ¼ cup chopped red onion

   2 tsp fajita or taco seasoning

   2 tsp olive oil (for cooking)

   2 whole-wheat tortillas

   1 tbsp reduced-fat sour cream

16 fl oz lemonade

Dinner

3 oz grilled chicken breast

   rubbed with 1 tsp mixed herbs

   basted with 1 tsp olive oil

1 whole-wheat dinner roll

1 cup chopped, steamed broccoli

1 medium baked potato with skin and topping

    3 tbsp reduced-fat sour cream

    2 tbsp reduced-fat, shredded cheddar cheese

    1 tbsp chopped tomatoes

    1 tsp bacon bits

    1 tsp chopped chives

    1 tbsp soft margarine spread

8 fl oz 100% fruit juice

1 small/medium piece angel food cake

Snacks

    10 oz nonfat milk

    1 oz gingersnaps (about 4 small cookies)

Nutrition Facts	Total kilocalories: 2,532	Grams of carbohydrates: 356
	Percent of calories from carbohydrates: 56	Grams of proteins: 115
	Percent of calories from proteins: 18	Grams of fats: 72
	Grams of saturated fats:17.4 (6%)	Grams of trans fats: 0
	Percent of calories from fats: 26	Grams of fiber: 31

Day 7

Breakfast

    2 4-inch pancakes, from frozen batter

    2 tbsp natural peanut butter (You can substitute almond butter, walnut butter, or soy-nut butter for peanut butter.)

    2 tbsp pancake syrup

    ½ cup fresh blueberries

    8 oz nonfat milk

Lunch

    Chicken soup with lentils (see recipe page 221)

    1 medium apple

    1 tbsp peanut butter (You can substitute almond butter, walnut butter, or soy-nut butter for peanut butter.)

Dinner

1 cup hearty vegetable soup (ready to serve from a can or homemade)

2 slices whole-wheat bread, toasted

1 tbsp apple butter

1 cup shredded hash browns cooked in 1 tbsp olive oil

6 oz broiled beef flank steak, lean

6 asparagus stalks

½ cup berry cobbler

Snacks

5 cups air-popped popcorn

Nutrition *Facts*	Total kilocalories: 2,496	Grams of carbohydrates: 308
	Percent of calories from carbohydrates: 50	Grams of proteins: 128
	Percent of calories from proteins: 20	Grams of fats: 84
	Grams of saturated fats: 18 (6%)	Grams of trans fats: 0
	Percent of calories from fats: 30	Grams of fiber: 40

Day 8

Breakfast

1 100% whole-wheat bagel

2 tbsp peanut butter (You can substitute almond butter, walnut butter, or soy-nut butter for peanut butter.)

2 tbsp fruit preserves

1 cup red grapes

1 tropical smoothie (see recipe page 222)

Lunch

1½ cups cooked whole-wheat spaghetti

¾ cup cooked, drained spinach

¾ diced, canned tomatoes

¾ cup steamed zucchini

1 Italian sausage link, cooked

1 tbsp olive oil

¼ cup part-skim mozzarella cheese

1 slice garlic bread

   1 slice toasted Italian bread

   2 tsp reduced-fat spread

   1 tsp fresh, minced garlic

Dinner

Breakfast for dinner

   1 Belgian waffle topped with

      ¼ cup sweet cherries in light syrup

   3 oz Canadian bacon

   6 oz light (reduced-sugar) yogurt topped with

      ½ cup low-fat granola (without raisins)

Snacks

10 oz nonfat milk

1 medium banana

Nutrition Facts	Total kilocalories: 2,515	Grams of carbohydrates: 373
	Percent of calories from carbohydrates: 59	Grams of proteins: 123
	Percent of calories from proteins: 20	Grams of fats: 59
	Grams of saturated fats: 21 (7.5%)	Grams of trans fats: 0
	Percent of calories from fats: 21	Grams of fiber: 33

Day 9

Breakfast

Fruit plate

   ½ cup each: cubed cantaloupe melon, cubed honeydew melon, diced
      pineapple, strawberries

½ cup low-fat granola (without raisins)

6 oz nonfat light (reduced-sugar) yogurt

Lunch

Rainbow burrito (see recipe page 222)

1 medium orange

1 PowerBar Protein Plus Bar

Dinner

2 cups tossed salad

3 tbsp fat-free French dressing

3 oz trout fillet
 tossed in 3 tbsp seasoned breading and cooked in 2 tsp olive oil

2 tbsp cocktail sauce

¾ cup green peas

1 cup deluxe light macaroni and cheese (Kraft)

½ cup fat-free chocolate pudding (snack cup)

Snacks

6 oz chocolate nonfat milk

½ cup dry-roasted pistachios

Nutrition Facts		
Total kilocalories: 2,484	Grams of carbohydrates: 354
Percent of calories from carbohydrates: 57	Grams of proteins: 114
Percent of calories from proteins: 19	Grams of fats: 68
Grams of saturated fats: 13.7 (5%)	Grams of trans fats: 0
Percent of calories from fats: 25	Grams of fiber: 37

Day 10

Breakfast

1 large, 100% whole-wheat bagel

2 tbsp natural peanut butter, chunky (You can substitute almond butter, walnut butter, or soy-nut butter for peanut butter.)

2 tbsp jam or preserves

1 cup fresh blueberries

12 oz cappuccino made with low-fat milk

Lunch

Pita packed with tuna salad
 1 whole-wheat pita

Tuna salad

    ½ cup tuna, canned in water, drained

    3 tbsp reduced-fat mayonnaise

    2 tsp Dijon mustard

    2 small dill pickles, chopped

    3 large green olives, chopped

    ¼ cup chopped green bell pepper

  2 leafs lettuce

  2 slices tomato

12 fl oz fresh-squeezed orange juice

Dinner

1 BBQ turkey burger (see recipe page 222)

1 whole-wheat roll

1 slice low-fat Swiss cheese

1 cup mixed greens

¼ cup diced tomato

1 tsp sesame oil

2 tsp seasoned rice vinegar

1 chocolate-banana smoothie:

1 medium banana (sliced and frozen)

¾ cup nonfat milk

2 tbsp chocolate syrup

4–5 ice cubes

Snacks

1 PowerBar Triple Threat Fusion Bar

8 oz pink lemonade drink

Nutrition Facts	Total kilocalories: 2,530	Grams of carbohydrates: 363
	Percent of calories from carbohydrates: 57	Grams of proteins: 112
	Percent of calories from proteins: 18	Grams of fats: 70
	Grams of saturated fats: 15.6 (5.5%)	Grams of trans fats: 0
	Percent of calories from fats: 25	Grams of fiber: 37

Day 11

Breakfast

1 medium banana

1 PowerBar Nut Naturals Bar

12 oz coffee or herbal tea mixed with 1 oz nonfat milk

Lunch

Gourmet grilled cheese

  2 slices whole-wheat bread

  1 oz Gouda cheese

  1 tbsp reduced-fat spread

1 cup lentil soup

10 baby carrots

1 medium Bartlett pear

6 fl oz chai tea made with soy milk

Dinner

Teriyaki salmon with roasted sweet potato fries (see recipe page 223)

1 cup steamed broccoli

1 cup mixed berries

½ cup nonfat vanilla yogurt

Snacks

8 whole-wheat saltine crackers

2 oz low-fat cheddar cheese

1 cup fruit cocktail canned in natural juices

Nutrition *Facts*	Total kilocalories: 2,523	Grams of carbohydrates: 326
	Percent of calories from carbohydrates: 52	Grams of proteins: 136
	Percent of calories from proteins: 22	Grams of fats: 75
	Grams of saturated fats: 17 (6%)	Grams of trans fats: 0
	Percent of calories from fats: 26	Grams of fiber: 36

Day 12

Breakfast

1 cup Cheerios cereal

10 oz nonfat milk

1 medium banana

1 cinnamon-raisin English muffin

1 tbsp soft spread

Lunch

Ultimate turkey sandwich (see recipe page 223)

1½ cups tomato vegetable soup

2 small oatmeal raisin cookies

Dinner

1 cup cooked cheese tortellini, tossed with

    ¾ cup marinara sauce

    2 garlic cloves

1 cup chopped fresh spinach, sautéed in

    1 tsp olive oil

3 oz grilled chicken breast

1 focaccia bread stick (from refrigerated dough)

Snack

Yogurt parfait

    1 cup nonfat vanilla yogurt

    ½ cup low-fat granola (without raisins)

    ½ cup sliced strawberries

    2 tbsp sliced almonds

Nutrition Facts		
Total kilocalories: 2,540	Grams of carbohydrates: 380	
Percent of calories from carbohydrates: 60	Grams of proteins: 120	
Percent of calories from proteins: 19	Grams of fats: 60	
Grams of saturated fats: 11 (4%)	Grams of trans fats: 0	
Percent of calories from fats: 21	Grams of fiber: 34	

Day 13

Breakfast

Breakfast sandwich made with

    1 egg white, cooked

    1 whole egg, cooked

    1 tsp vegetable spread

    2 slices whole-wheat toast

    1 slice low-fat (2% milk) American cheese

10 oz cappuccino made with low-fat milk

Lunch

Salad

    2 cups chopped romaine lettuce

    2 cups chopped red leaf lettuce

    2 tbsp sun-dried tomatoes

    3 pieces artichoke hearts, canned in water

    3 oz chopped Canadian bacon

    3 oz grilled chicken breast

    1 tbsp grated Parmesan cheese

    2 tbsp reduced-calorie Italian dressing

2 focaccia bread sticks made from refrigerated dough

1 snack pack of fat-free vanilla pudding

1 small banana

Dinner

1 whole-wheat pita bread, sliced and filled with

    3 falafel patties, each 2.5" in diameter

    6 slices cucumber

    4 slices tomato

    2 oz soft goat cheese

1 cup light vanilla ice cream

¼ cup dried plums

Snacks

1 PowerBar Pria Complete Nutrition Bar

1 fresh medium peach

16 oz green tea with 1 tbsp honey

Nutrition *Facts*	Total kilocalories: 2,453	Grams of carbohydrates: 320
	Percent of calories from carbohydrates: 53	Grams of proteins: 129
	Percent of calories from proteins: 20	Grams of fats: 73
	Grams of saturated fats: 26 (10%)	Grams of trans fats: 0
	Percent of calories from fats: 27	Grams of fiber: 29

Day 14

Breakfast

French toast made with

   3 slices 100% whole-wheat bread

   1 large egg mixed with 4 oz nonfat milk

   1 tbsp reduced-fat spread

   2 tbsp reduced-calorie pancake syrup

6 oz nonfat, light (reduced-sugar) yogurt

1 medium banana

Lunch

Taco salad

   1 whole-wheat tortilla

   3 cups chopped lettuce

   ¼ avocado

   ¼ cup sweet corn

   ¼ cup chopped tomatoes

   ¼ cup salsa

   ¼ cup shredded low-fat cheddar cheese

   1 cup vegetarian refried beans

   ¾ cup prepared Spanish rice

   2 tbsp reduced-fat sour cream

Dinner

Peanut butter stir fry with shrimp (see recipe page 224)

1 cup fruit sorbet

Snacks

1 Double Chocolate Crisp PowerBar Harvest Bar

Nutrition Facts	Total kilocalories: 2,483	Grams of carbohydrates: 378
	Percent of calories from carbohydrates: 61	Grams of proteins: 101
	Percent of calories from proteins: 16	Grams of fats: 63
	Grams of saturated fats: 11 (4%)	Grams of trans fats: 0
	Percent of calories from fats: 23	Grams of fiber: 38

The Energy to Burn Diet: 2,500-Calorie Recipes

QUINOA SALAD

Serves: 1

Cook Time: 15 minutes

Prep Time: 25 minutes

¼ cup quinoa, dry
½ cup water
½ cup cannelloni beans (rinsed and drained)
¼ cup diced red bell pepper
¼ cup chopped celery
¼ cup corn kernels

1 ½ tsp walnut oil
2 tsp seasoned rice vinegar
2 Tbs crumbled feta cheese
Salt and pepper to taste
2 cups chopped romaine lettuce
4 tortilla chips, crushed

Rinse and drain quinoa. In a small saucepan, combine quinoa and water, cover. Bring to a boil, reduce heat and simmer for 12–15 minutes, until water is absorbed and quinoa is tender.

Transfer cooked quinoa to a bowl and set aside to cool for at least 10 minutes or store in the refrigerator until needed.

In a medium bowl, combine cooked quinoa, cannelloni beans, bell pepper, celery, and corn.

Add walnut oil and vinegar, season with salt and pepper to taste; toss well to combine.

Add feta and serve over a bed of lettuce topped with crushed tortilla chips.

HOMEMADE LASAGNA

Serves: 6
Prep Time: 30 minutes
Cook Time: 50 minutes

10 oz (10 sheets) dry lasagna pasta
1 Tbs olive oil
8 oz raw ground chicken breast
2 clove garlic, minced
1 tsp red pepper flakes (optional)
1 tsp dried oregano
½ tsp kosher salt
1 cup canned tomato sauce

2 cups sliced zucchini
3 cups chopped raw spinach (stems removed)
1 cup part skim ricotta cheese
1 cup finely shredded part skim mozzarella cheese
¼ cup grated parmesan cheese
Nonstick cooking spray

Preheat oven to 375°F.

Fill a large bowl with very hot tap water. Add pasta to bowl, set aside and allow to soak for 20 minutes.

While the pasta is soaking, heat oil in a sauce pan over medium heat.

Add chicken and sauté for 3–5 minutes until lightly browned.

Add garlic, red pepper, oregano, salt, and tomato sauce; stir to combine and bring to a simmer.

Add zucchini and spinach and continue to simmer for an additional 5 minutes until zucchini is tender. Turn off heat and set aside.

Drain pasta.

Spray a large rectangular baking dish with cooking spray and spread ¼ of the chicken mixture in the bottom of the dish.

Lay 4 sheets of pasta in the bottom of the dish. Gently spoon ¼ cup (12 teaspoons) of ricotta cheese evenly on top of the pasta.

Layer another ¼ of the chicken mixture and top with ¼ cup of mozzarella cheese.

For the next layer, place 3 sheets of pasta, followed by another ¼ cup ricotta cheese, ¼ more chicken mixture, and an additional ¼ cup mozzarella.

Layer the last 3 sheets of pasta followed by remaining ricotta, chicken mixture, and mozzarella.

Sprinkle top of lasagna with grated parmesan cheese.

Cover with aluminum foil and bake for 35 minutes.

Remove foil and continue to cook for an additional 15 minutes until cheese is melted and bubbly.

Allow to cool for 10 minutes before serving.

MACARONI AND CHEESE

Serves: 1
Cook Time: 15–20 minutes
Prep Time: 5–10 minutes

1½ cup cooked, whole-wheat macaroni (about ⅔ cup dry noodles)

½ cup shredded, low-fat cheddar cheese
½ cup 1% milk

Bring 4–5 cups of water to a boil in a medium-sized saucepan.

Add macaroni to pan, return to a low boil, and cook noodles until al dente, about 15–20 minutes.

While macaroni is cooking, heat milk in a small saucepan over medium heat.

Bring milk to a simmer and add low-fat cheddar cheese. Continue to cook over medium heat, stirring constantly, until cheese has melted.

When macaroni reaches preferred consistency, drain and return to pan. Pour cheese mixture over macaroni and toss evenly to coat.

Serve with broccoli on the side or toss with cooked broccoli as desired.

ROASTED VEGETABLES WITH BROWN RICE PASTA

Serves: 1
Cook Time: 15 minutes
Prep Time: 10 minutes

1 clove garlic, chopped
1 cup chopped broccoli
½ cup grape or cherry tomatoes
1 cup sliced mushrooms
¼ cup shelled soybeans (edamame)
2 tsp olive oil

1 tsp balsamic vinegar
2 oz dry brown rice
2 Tbs low-fat plain yogurt (Greek-style yogurt preferred)
¼ cup fresh parsley, chopped
Salt and pepper to taste

Preheat oven to 400°F.

Place garlic, broccoli, tomatoes, mushrooms, and soybeans on a baking sheet.

Season with oil, vinegar, salt, and pepper; roast for 10–12 minutes until vegetables are just tender.

Cook pasta according to package directions, drain.

In a large bowl, combine roasted vegetables, cooked pasta, yogurt, and parsley; toss to combine and serve.

QUICK & EASY SALAD

Serves: 1
Cook Time: 0 minutes
Prep Time: 5 minutes

1 tsp seasoned rice vinegar
2 tsp extra virgin olive oil
¼ tsp Dijon mustard

Lemon juice to taste
2 cups mixed greens

In a small salad bowl add vinegar, oil, mustard, and a squeeze of lemon juice; whisk well to combine.

Add greens to bowl, toss to coat with dressing, and serve.

TOMATO & BASIL PIZZA

Serves: 1
Cook Time: 15 minutes
Prep Time: 10 minutes

1 (6 in) whole wheat pita bread
1 plum tomato, sliced
5 fresh basil leaves
1 thin slice red onion (separate rings)

¼ cup shredded part skim mozzarella cheese
½ tsp dried oregano
2 tsp olive oil

Preheat oven to 400°F.

Place pita bread on a baking sheet lined with aluminum foil.

Top with tomato, basil, onion, and cheese.

Sprinkle with oregano, drizzle with oil, and bake for 10–12 minutes until cheese is melted and bubbly.

SALAD WITH WALNUT DRESSING

Serves: 1
Cook Time: 0 minutes
Prep Time: 5 minutes

1 tsp red wine vinegar
2 tsp walnut oil
¼ tsp Dijon mustard

Lemon juice to taste
2 cups mixed greens

In a small salad bowl add vinegar, oil, mustard, and a squeeze of lemon juice; whisk well to combine.

Add greens to bowl, toss to coat with dressing, and serve.

MEXICAN TORTILLA BAKE

Serves: 2
Cook Time: 25 minutes
Prep Time: 15 minutes

1 tsp olive oil
½ pound ground chicken breast
½ small onion, diced
1 clove garlic, minced
1 tsp cumin
1 tsp chili powder
½ zucchini, sliced
1 yellow bell pepper, chopped
½ jalapeno pepper, minced
(optional)

3 whole wheat flour tortillas
½ avocado
½ cup shredded low fat cheddar
cheese
¾ cup salsa (¼ cup for filling,
¼ cup for topping, ¼ cup to
mix with avocado)
Salt and pepper to taste
Nonstick cooking spray

Preheat oven to 375°.

Heat olive oil in a large skillet, add chicken, and sauté for 2–3 minutes until slightly browned.

Add onion and garlic; cook for an additional 2 minutes.

Season with salt, pepper, cumin, and chili powder, stir to combine.

Add zucchini, bell pepper, and jalapeno and cook, stirring continuously until chicken is no longer pink and vegetables are slightly tender.

Turn off heat and set skillet aside.

Spray a 9-inch pie plate or square casserole dish with non-stick spray.

Place one flour tortilla on the bottom of the pan, top with half of the chicken mixture, ½ cup salsa, and 2 Tbs cheese.

Create second layer with another tortilla, remaining chicken, and 2 Tbs of cheese.

Create top layer with remaining tortilla, ¼ cup salsa, and remaining cheese.

Transfer to oven and bake until cheese is melted (about 15 minutes).

Slice and serve with diced avocado mixed with remaining ¼ cup salsa.

CHICKEN SOUP WITH LENTILS

Serves: 1
Cook Time: 15 minutes
Prep Time: 5 minutes

2 cups low-sodium chicken broth
1.5 oz dry whole-wheat penne
pasta
½ cup frozen green peas and carrots
⅓ cup canned lentils (rinsed and
drained)

3 oz grilled chicken breast,
shredded
1 tsp extra virgin olive oil
Salt and pepper to taste

In a small saucepan bring chicken broth to a boil.

Add pasta and cook for 8 minutes.

Add peas and carrots, lentils, and shredded chicken; continue to cook until pasta is tender.

Transfer to a bowl, top with olive oil, and serve.

TROPICAL SMOOTHIE
Serves: 1
Prep Time: 5 minutes
Cook Time: 0 minutes

½ medium banana
½ cup frozen pineapple chunks
4 large strawberries, sliced

2 Tbs non fat vanilla yogurt
½ cup freshly squeezed orange juice
¼ cup water

Combine ingredients in a blender; blend until smooth.

RAINBOW BURRITO
Serves: 1
Cook Time: 1 minute
Prep Time: 5 minutes

1 (8 in) whole wheat flour tortilla
½ cup cooked long-grain brown rice
¼ cup canned black beans (rinsed
  and drained)

¼ cup baby spinach leaves
2 Tbs salsa
2 Tbs diced avocado

Top tortilla with rice, beans, spinach, salsa, and avocado; wrap tightly.
Microwave for 30–60 seconds on high heat.

BBQ TURKEY BURGER
Makes 4 burgers
Cook Time: 10 minutes
Prep Time: 10 minutes

1 pound ground turkey breast
¼ cup finely chopped red onion
½ cup chopped mushrooms
½ cup seasoned breadcrumbs
2 Tbs light mayonnaise

2 Tbs barbeque sauce
¼ cup chopped fresh basil
¼ tsp salt
Black pepper to taste

Preheat grill or skillet to medium.
Combine ingredients in a large bowl.

Mix well and form into 4 equal sized burgers.

Cook burgers for 4–5 minutes per side or until completely cooked.

TERIYAKI SALMON WITH ROASTED SWEET POTATO FRIES

Serves: 1

Cook Time: 45 minutes

Prep Time: 15 minutes (plus 30 minutes to marinate)

1 large sweet potato	1 Tbs honey
2 tsp canola oil	1 tsp grated fresh ginger root
2 Tbs reduced sodium soy sauce	1 clove garlic, minced
1 tsp sesame oil	½ tsp hot sauce to taste
1 Tbs lime juice	5 oz wild salmon

Preheat oven to 425°.

Scrub sweet potato well and cut into ½-in thick fries (do not peel).

Transfer fries to a bowl of cold water and soak for 5 minutes.

Remove from water, dry fries very well with a clean dish towel, and distribute evenly on a large baking sheet.

Season with salt and pepper; roast potatoes for about 35 minutes or until golden brown, turning once.

While the potatoes are cooking, prepare the salmon. For the marinade, in a small bowl combine, soy sauce, sesame oil, lime juice, honey, ginger, garlic, and hot sauce.

Place salmon in a resealable bag, add marinade, and refrigerate for 20 minutes.

Preheat grill or grill pan.

Grill salmon for 4–5 minutes per side or until cooked through. Serve with sweet potato fries.

ULTIMATE TURKEY SANDWICH

Serves: 1

Cook Time: 0 minutes

Prep Time: 5 minutes

2 slices whole grain bread, toasted	¼ cup baby spinach leaves
1 Tbs hummus	¼ yellow or red bell pepper, sliced
3 oz sliced roasted turkey breast	1 thin slice red onion
1 slice low-fat Swiss cheese	

Spread hummus in an even layer on one slice of bread.

Top with turkey, cheese, spinach, pepper, onion, and remaining slice of bread.

PEANUT BUTTER STIR FRY WITH SHRIMP

Serves: 1
Cook Time: 15 minutes
Prep Time: 10 minutes

¼ cup dry long-grain brown rice
2 tsp canola oil
4 oz raw, large shrimp, peeled and
  de-veined
1 clove garlic, minced
1 inch piece ginger root, minced
1 cup chopped broccoli

1 cup baby spinach leaves
½ cup chopped carrot
¼ red onion chopped
1 Tbsp reduced sodium soy sauce
1 Tbsp creamy peanut butter
Juice of ½ lime

Prepare brown rice according to package directions, set aside.

Heat oil in pan or wok over medium-high heat, add ginger and garlic, sauté for 15 seconds.

Add shrimp, cook for 1–2 minutes.

Add broccoli, spinach, and carrots, toss.

Add soy sauce and lime juice. Toss and continue to cook, tossing continuously for 2–3 minutes.

Add peanut butter. Continue to toss and cook until shrimp is fully cooked and vegetables are crisp-tender.

Add cooked brown rice, toss, and serve.

The Energy to Burn Diet: 2,500-Calorie Grocery List

Beverages

100% fruit juice, any variety
Coffee
Lemonade
Orange juice, freshly squeezed
Tea, chai
Tea, herbal
Tea, green

Bread and Grains

Bread products
  Bagel, 100% whole-wheat
  Dinner roll, Parker House
    variety

Dinner roll, whole-wheat
English muffin, 100% whole-
  wheat
Italian bread
Pita bread, whole-wheat
Sandwich bread, 100% whole-
  wheat
Sandwich bread, whole-grain
Tortilla, whole-wheat
Garlic Parmesan bread sticks
  (from refrigerated dough)
Focaccia bread sticks (from
  refrigerated dough)
Rice, pasta, other grains

Lasagna noodles
Macaroni noodles, whole-wheat
Penne, whole-wheat
Spaghetti, whole-wheat
Rice, brown
Rice, wild
Rice, boxed, Spanish variety
Quinoa

Cereals

Granola, low-fat, without
  raisins
Oatmeal, steel-cut or
  old-fashioned
Wheat-bran flakes

Fruits

Apple, any variety
Banana
Berries, mixed
Blueberries
Cranberries, dried
Grapes, red
Lime
Mango
Melon, cantaloupe
Melon, honeydew
Papaya
Peach
Pears, Bartlett
Pineapple (canned)
Plums, dried
Raisins

Raisins, golden
Strawberries

Vegetables

Asparagus
Avocado
Broccoli, fresh or frozen
Bell pepper, green
Bell pepper, red
Bell pepper, yellow
Carrots, baby
Celery
Cucumber
Corn (canned)
Edamame (fresh soybeans)
Garlic
Green beans, haricot vert or
  canned
Jalapeño pepper
Lettuce
Mixed greens
Mushrooms, fresh, any variety
Onion, red
Onion, yellow
Potato, russet or Idaho
Potato, sweet
Red leaf lettuce
Romaine lettuce
Spinach, baby
Tomatoes, grape or cherry variety
Tomatoes, plum variety
Tomatoes, sun-dried
Zucchini

Dairy Products and Milk Substitutes

Milk, nonfat (skim)

Milk, 1% milk fat

Cheeses

Cottage cheese, low-fat

American, low-fat, slices

Cheddar cheese, low-fat, shredded

Feta cheese, crumbled

Goat cheese

Gouda

Mozzarella cheese, part-skim, shredded

Parmesan cheese, grated

Ricotta cheese, part-skim

Swiss cheese, low-fat

Sour cream, reduced-fat

Yogurt, nonfat, light (reduced-sugar)

Yogurt, nonfat (fruit on the bottom)

Yogurt, Greek-style, plain

Meat and Poultry

Eggs

Beef, flank steak

Bacon, Canadian

Chicken, boneless, skinless breast, fresh

Chicken, boneless, skinless breast, ground

Pork tenderloin

Pork sausage, Italian, link

Turkey breast, ground

Turkey breast, deli meat

Beans, Legumes, Alternate Protein Sources

Beans, cannelloni (canned)

Beans, black (canned)

Beans, vegetarian, refried

Nuts

Pistachios

Walnuts

Seafood

Salmon, fillet

Shrimp, ready to serve, fresh or frozen

Trout, fillet

Tuna, canned in water

Fats and Oils

Butter spray, noncalorie

Peanut butter, creamy natural; you can substitute almond butter, walnut butter, or soy-nut butter for peanut butter

Vegetable spread, reduced-fat

Vegetable spread, regular

Canola oil

Olive oil

Sesame oil

Walnut oil

Canned Foods

Artichoke hearts

Chicken broth, low-sodium

Cherries (pie filling) in light syrup

Corn

Cranberry relish

Fruit cocktail, light or in its own juices

Lentils

Mushrooms

Tomato sauce

Tomatoes, diced

Soup (select low-sodium when able)

  Hot and sour Chinese soup

  Hearty vegetable soup

  Lentil soup

  Minestrone soup

  Tomato vegetable soup

Frozen Foods

Belgian waffles

Pancakes, approx. 4" in diameter

Potatoes, hash brown or shredded

Vegetables, green peas and carrots mix

Vegetables, mixed

Sorbet, citrus flavor

Frozen yogurt, nonfat, vanilla

Snack Foods

Animal crackers

Crackers, whole-wheat saltines

Popcorn, air-popped

PowerBar products

  PowerBar Nut Naturals Bar

  PowerBar Pria 110 Plus Bar

  PowerBar Pria Complete Nutrition Bar

  PowerBar Protein Plus Bar

Pretzels, whole-wheat

Rice cakes, mini, any flavor

Tortilla chips

Desserts

Angel food cake

Berry cobbler, from bakery

Fig cookies

Gingersnaps, small

Oatmeal raisin cookies, small

Pudding, snack pack, low-fat

Convenience Foods

Macaroni and cheese (deluxe), light; we recommend Kraft deluxe macaroni and cheese dinner, light

Tortellini, cheese

Falafel patties, 2½" in diameter

Condiments, Helpers, and Baking Products

Apple butter

Bacon bits

Barbeque sauce

Bread crumbs, seasoned

Cocktail sauce

Fruit preserves or jam, 100% fruit

Honey

Hot sauce

Hummus, any variety

Lemon juice

Lime juice

Marinara sauce

Mayonnaise, reduced-fat

Mustard, Dijon
Nonstick cooking spray
Olives, green
Pickles, dill
Salad dressings
  Caesar, fat-free
  French, fat-free
  Italian, reduced-fat
Salsa, any variety
Soy sauce, reduced-sodium
Sugar, brown
Syrup
  Chocolate, fat-free
  Maple
  Pancake

Pancake, reduced-calorie
Vinegar, balsamic
Vinegar, rice wine

Seasonings
Basil, fresh (preferred)
Chili powder
Cumin
Chives, fresh or dried
Fajita (taco) seasoning
Ginger root, fresh, grated
Oregano, flakes
Parsley, fresh (preferred)
Pepper, black and red
Salt, kosher and iodized

Selected Readings

Chapter 1. Nutrition Condition

Dietary Guidelines for Americans, 6th ed., Home and Garden Bulletin No. 232. Washington, D.C.: U.S. Government Printing Office, 2005.

Drewnoski A. Concept of a Nutritious Food: Toward a Nutrient Density Score. *Am J Clin Nutr* 2005; 82:721–732.

Economos CD, Bortz SS, Nelson ME. Nutritional practices of elite athletes. Practical recommendation. *Sports Med* 1993;16(6):381–399.

Fogli-Cawely JJ, Dwyer JT, Saltzman E et al. The 2005 Dietary Guidelines for Americans Adherence Index: development and application. *J Nutr* 2006;136(11)2908–2915.

Labouze E, Goffi C, Moulay L et al. A multipurpose tool to evaluate the nutritional quality of individual foods: Nutrimap. *Public Health Nutr* 2007;10(7):690–700.

Ostry A, Young ML, Hughes M. The quality of nutritional information available on popular websites: a content analysis. *Health Educ Res* 2007. Accessed October 9, 2007: doi:10.1093/her/cym050.

Phillips SM. Dietary protein for athletes: from requirements to metabolic advantage. *Appl Physiol Nutr Metab* 2006;6:647–654.

Position of the American Dietetic Association, Dietitians of Canada, and American College of Sports Medicine: Nutrition and Athletic Performance. *J Am Diet Assoc* 2000;100: 1543–1556.

Tipton KD, Wolfe, RR. Protein and amino acids for athletes. *J Sports Sci* 2004;22:65–79.

Williams C. Dietary macro- and micronutrient requirements of endurance athletes *Proc Nutr Soc* 1998; 57:1–8.

Chapter 2. Your Perfect Weight

Anderson GH, Moore SE. Dietary proteins in the regulation of food intake and body weight in humans. *J Nutr* 2004;134:974S–979S.

Cureton KJ, Sparling PB. Distance running performance and metabolic responses to running in men and women with excess weight experimentally equated. *Med Sci Sports Exerc* 1980;2:288–294.

Cureton KJ, Sparling PB, Evans BW et al. Effect of experimental alterations in excess weight on aerobic capacity and distance running performance. *Med Sci Sports* 1978;10:194–199.

Doi T, Matsuo T, Sugawara M et al. New approach for weight reduction by a combination of diet, light resistance exercise and the timing of ingesting a protein supplement. *Asia Pac J Clin Nutr* 2001;10(3):275–285.

Esmarck B, Andersen JL, Olsen S. et al. Timing of postexercise protein intake is important for muscle hypertrophy with resistance training in elderly humans. *J Phys* 2001;535(1):301–311.

Feinman RD, Fine EJ: Thermodynamics and metabolic advantage of weight loss diets. *Metab Syn Relat* Dis. 2003;1:209–219.

Hill JH, Blundell JE. Macronutrients and satiety: The effects of a high-protein or high-carbohydrate meal on subjective motivation to eat and food preferences. *Nutr Behav* 1986; 3:133–144.

Janssen I, Katzmarzyk PT, Ross R. Waist circumference and not body mass index explains obesity-related health risk. *Am J Clin Nutr* 2004 Mar;79(3):379–384.

Layman D. Protein quality and quantity at levels above the RDA improves adult weight loss. *J Amer Coll Nutr* 2004;23(9):631S–636S.

Layman DK et al. Dietary protein and exercise have additive effects on body composition during weight loss in adult women. *Amer Soc Nutr Sci J Nutr* 2005;135:1903–1910.

Layman DK, Boileau RA, Erickson DJ et al. A reduced ratio of dietary carbohydrate to protein improves body composition and blood lipid profiles during weight loss in adult women. *J Nutr* 2003;133:411–417.

Marks BL, Ward A, Morris DH et al. Fat-free mass is maintained in women following a moderate diet and exercise program. *Med Sci Sport Exer* 1995;27(9):1243–1251.

Rankin JW, Shute M, Heffron SP et al. Energy restriction but not protein affects antioxidant capacity in athletes. *Free Radic Biol Med* 2006;41(6):1001–9.

Rasmussen BB, Tipton KD, Miller SL, Wolf SE, Wolfe RR. An oral essential amino acid-carbohydrate supplement enhances muscle protein anabolism after resistance exercise. *J Appl Physiol* 2000;88:386–392.

Ross R, Pedwell H, Rossanen J. Response of total and regional lean tissue and skeletal muscle to a program of energy restriction and resistance exercise. *Intl J Ob.*

Roza AM, Shizgal HM. The Harris-Benedict equation reevaluated: resting energy requirements and body cell mass. *Am J Clin Nutr* 1984;40:168–182.

Tipton KD, Ferrando AA, Phillips SM, Doyle D Jr, Wolfe RR. Postexercise net protein synthesis in human muscle from orally administered amino acids. *Am J Physiol Endocrinol Metab* 1999;276:E628–E634.

Tipton KD, Ferrando AA, Williams BD, Wolfe RR. Muscle protein metabolism in female swimmers after a combination of resistance and endurance exercise. *J Appl Physiol* 1996; 81:2034–2038.

Tipton KD, Gurkin BE, Matin S, Wolfe RR. Nonessential amino acids are not necessary to stimulate net muscle protein synthesis in healthy volunteers. *J Nutr Biochem* 1999;10:89–95.

Tipton KD, Rasmussen BB, Miller SL, Wolf SE, Owens-Stovall SK, Petrini BE, Wolfe RR. Timing of amino acid-carbohydrate ingestion alters anabolic response of muscle to resistance exercise. *Am J Physiol Endocrinol Metab* 2001;281:E197–E206.

Tipton KD, Wolfe RR. Exercise-induced changes in protein metabolism. *Acta Physiol Scand* 1998;162:377–387.

Zhu, S. et al. Race-ethnicity-specific waist circumference cutoffs for identifying cardiovascular disease risk factors. *Am J Clin Nutr* 2005 81: 409–415.

Chapter 3. Carbohydrates

American College of Sports Medicine. Position stand on exercise and fluid replacement. *Med Sci Sport Exerc* 1996;28:i–vii.

Brand, MJ. et al. *The G.I. Factor: The Glycaemic Index Solution.* Sydney, Australia: Hodder & Stoughton, 1996.

Burke LM et al. Guidelines for carbohydrate intake: Do athletes achieve them? *Sports Med* 2001;31(4):267–299. Review.

Burke LM et al. Muscle glycogen storage after prolonged exercise: effect of the glycemic index of carbohydrate feedings. *J App Physiol* l993;75:1019–1023.

Burke, LM, Hawley JA. Effects of short-term fat adaptation on metabolism and performance of prolonged exercise. *Med Sci Sports Exerc* 2002;34(9):1492–1498. Review.

Clark, N. Carb-loading tips for endurance athletes. *Amer Fitness*2007;25(2): 26–27.

Dunford, M. Carbohydrate and Exercise. In *Sports Nutrition: A Practice Manual for Professionals*, 4th ed.Chicago: American Dietetic Association, 2006, 14–32.

———. Nutrition for Endurance Sports. In *Sports Nutrition: A Practice Manual for Professionals*, 4th ed. Chicago: American Dietetic Association, 2006, 445–459.

Frayn, K. *Metabolic Regulation: A Human Perspective*, 2nd ed. Blackwell, 2003.

Jeukendrup AE, Jentjens RL, Moseley L. Nutritional considerations in triathlon. *Sports Med* 2005;35(2):163–181.

Joint Position Statement of American College of Sports Medicine, American Dietetic Association and Dietitians of Canada. Nutrition and Athletic Performance. *Med Sci Sports Exerc* 2000;32(12), 2130–2145.

Kushner RF, Doerfler B. Low-carbohydrate, high-protein diets revisited. *Curr Opin Gastroenterol* 2008;24(2):198–203. Review.

Rosenkranz RR, Cook CM, Haub MD. *Int J of Sports Nutr Exerc Metab* 2007; 17(13), 296–309.

Whitney EN, Sharon RR. *Understanding Nutrition*, 9th ed. Belmont, Calif: Wadsworth, 2002.

Chapter 4. Proteins

American College of Sports Medicine, American Dietetic Association, Dietitians of Canada. Joint Position Statement: Nutrition and Athletic Performance. *Med Sci Sports Exerc* 2000;32:2130–2145.

Aronson D. Vegetarian nutrition: what every dietitian should know. *Today's Dietitian* 2005;7(3):32.

Charge SBP, Rudnicki MA. Cellular and molecular regulation of muscle regeneration. *Physiol Rev* 2004;84:209–238.

Dunford M. *Sports Nutrition: A Practice Manual for Professionals*, 4th ed. Chicago: American Dietetic Association, 2006.

Duyff RL. *The American Dietetic Association's Complete Food & Nutrition Guide*. Minneapolis: Chronimed, 1998.

Jentjens RL et al. Addition of protein and amino acids to carbohydrate does not enhance postexercise muscle glycogen synthesis. *J Appl Physiol* 2001;91(2):839–846.

Koopman, R et al. Combined ingestion of protein and free leucine with carbohydrate increases postexercise muscle protein synthesis in vivo in male subjects. *AJP Endo* 2005;288:645–653.

Nemet D et al. Proteins and amino acid supplementation in sports: are they truly necessary? *IMAJ*; 2005;7:328–332.

Phillips, SM. Dietary protein for athletes: from requirements to metabolic advantage. *Appl Physiol Nutr Metab* 2006;31:647–654.

———. Protein requirements and supplementation in strength sports. *Nutrition* 2004;20: 689–695.

Rasmussen RB, Phillips SM. Contractile and nutritional regulation of human muscle growth. *Exerc Sport Sci Rev* 2003;31(3):127–131.

Rennie MJ, Tipton KD. Protein and amino acid metabolism during and after exercise and the effects of nutrition. *Annu Rev Nutrition* 2000;20:457–483.

Tarnopolsky, M. Protein requirements for endurance athletes. *Nutrition* 2004;20:662–668.

Thompson J, Manore M. Proteins: crucial components of all body tissues. In *Nutrition: An Applied Approach*, MyPyramid ed. San Francisco: Benjamin Cummings, 2006.

Tipton KD, Wolfe RR. Exercise, protein metabolism, and muscle growth. *Int J SportNutr Exerc Metab* 2001;11:109–132.

Van Loon LJC et al. Maximizing postexercise muscle glycogen synthesis: carbohydrate supplementation and the application of amino acid or protein hydrolysate mixtures. *Am J Clin Nutr* 2000;72:106–111.

Wildman R, Miller B. *Sports and Fitness Nutrition*. Thomson Wadsworth. 2004.

Willoughby DS et al. Effects of resistance training and protein plus amino acid supplementation on muscle anabolism, mass, and strength. *Amino Acids* 2007;32:467–477.

Wolinsky I, ed. *Nutrition in Exercise and Sport*, 3rd ed. Boca Raton, Fla.: CRC Press, 1998.

Chapter 5. Fats for Life

American College of Sports Medicine and American Dietetic Association. Joint Position Statement: Nutrition and Athletic Performance. *Med. Sci. Sports Exerc* 2000;32; 12:2130–2145.

Burke LM, Deakin V. *Clinical Sports Nutrition*, 3rd ed. Sydney, Australia: McGraw-Hill, 2006.

Burke LM, Kiens B, Ivy JL. Carbohydrates and fat for training and recovery. *J Sports Sci* 2004;22:15–30.

Chanmugam P, Guthrie JF et al. Did fat intake in the United States really decline between 1989-1991 and 1994-1996? *JADA* 2003;103(7):867–872.

Dunford M. *Sports Nutrition: A Practice Manual for Professionals*, 4th ed. Chicago: American Dietetic Association, 2006.

Duyff RL, ed., *American Dietetic Association Complete Food and Nutrition Guide*, 2nd ed. Hoboken, N.J.: John Wiley & Sons, 2002, 52–73.

Institute of Medicine. *Dietary Reference Intakes for Energy, Carbohydrate, Fiber, Fat, Fatty Acids, Cholesterol, Protein and Amino Acids*. Washington, D.C.: National Academy Press, 2002.

Ranallo RF, Rhodes EC. Lipid metabolism during exercise. *Sports Med* 1990;26:29–42.

Rosenbloom C. *Sports Nutrition: A Guide for the Professional Working with Active People*, 3rd ed. Chicago: American Dietetic Association, 1999.

Votruba SB, Atkinson RL et al. Prior exercise increases subsequent utilization of dietary fat. *Med. Sci. Sports Exerc* 2002;34 (11):1757–1765.

Chapter 6. Energize

Coyle EF, et al. Substrated usage during prolonged exercise following a preexercise meal. *J Appl Physiol* 1985;59:429–433.

DeMarco HM, et al. The pre-exercise carbohydrate meals: application of glycemic index. *MSSE* 1999;31(1):164–170.

Febbraio MA, et al. Preexercise carbohydrate ingestion, glucose kinetics, and muscle glycogen use: effect of the glycemic index. *J Appl Physiol* 2000;89:1845–1851.

Goforth HW et al. Persistence of supercompensated muscle glycogen in trained subjects after carbohydrate loading. *J Appl Physiol* 1997;82:342–347.

Jeukendrup AE et al. Nutritional Considerations in Triathlon. *Sports Med* 2005;35(2):163–181.

Kundrat S. *101 Sports Nutrition Tips*. Monterey, Calif.: Coaches Choice, 2005.

Neufer PD et al. Improvements in exercise performance: effects of carbohydrate feedings and diet. *J Ap Phys* 1987;62:983–988.

Position of the American Dietetic Association, Dietitians of Canada, and American College of Sports Medicine. Nutrition and Athletic Performance. *J Am Diet Assoc* 2000;100: 1543–1556.

Sawka MN et al. American College of Sports Medicine Position Stand: Exercise and Fluid Replacement. www.acsm-msse.org, 2007.

Schabort EJ, Bosch AN, Weltan SM, Noaker TD. The effect of a preexercise meal on time to fatigue during prolonged cycling exercise. *MSSE* 1999;31(3):464–471.

Sherman WM, Brodowicz G, Wright DA, Allen WK, Wimonsen J, Dernbach A. Effects of 4 hour pre-exercise carbohydrate feedings on cycling performance. *MSSE* 1989;21:598–604.

Sherman WM, Peden MC, Wright DA. Carbohydrate feedings 1 hour before exercise improves cycling performance. *AJCN* 1991;54:866–870.

Tarnopolsky M. Protein requirements for endurance athletes. *Nutrition* 2004;20:663–668.

Williams C, Serratosa L. Nutrition on match day. *J Sports Sci* 2006;24(7):687–697.

Wu CL, Williams C. A low glycemic index meal before exercise improves running capacity in men. *J Sports Nutr Exer Metab* 2006;40:363–366.

Chapter 7. On the Go

Adopo E, Peronnet F, Massicotte D et al. Respective oxidation of exogenous glucose and fructose in the same drink during exercise. *J Appl Physiol* 1994;76:1014–1019.

American College of Sports Medicine. Position stand on exercise and fluid replacement. *Med Sci Sport Exerc* 1996;28:i–vii.

Bergeron MF, Armstrong LE, Maresh LE. Fluid and electrolyte losses during tennis in the heat. *Clin Sports Med* 1995;14:23–33.

Bergeron MF, Maresh CF, Armstrong, LE et al. Fluid-electrolyte balance associated with tennis match play in a hot environment. *Int J Sport Nutr* 1995;5:180–193.

Currell K, Jeukendrup A. Superior endurance performance with ingestion of multiple transportable carbohydrates. *Med Sci Sports Exerc* 2008;40:275–281.

Gisolfo CV, Summers RW, Schedl HP, Bleiler TL. Intestinal water absorption from select carbohydrate solutions in humans. *J Appl Physiol* 1992;73:2142–2150.

Jeukendrup AE, Jentjens R. Oxidation of carbohydrate feedings during prolonged exercise. *Sports Med* 2000;29:407–424.

Jeukendrup AE, Jentjens RL, Moseley L. Nutritional considerations in triathlon. *Sports Med* 2005;35(2):163–181.

Jeukendrup AE, Moseley L et al. Exogenous carbohydrate oxidation during ultraendurance exercise. *J Appl Physiol* 100:1134–1141.

Mack GW, Nose H, Nadel ER. Role of cardiopulmonary baroreflexes during dynamic exercise. *J Appl Physiol* 1988;65:1827–1832.

Maughan RJ, Leiper JB, Shirreffs SM. Rehydration and recovery after exercise. *Sport Sci Exch* 1996;9(62):1–5.

Nose H, Mack GW, Shi X et al. Role of osmolality and plasma volume during rehydration in humans. *J Appl Physiol* 1988;65:325–331.

Peters HP, Bos M, Seebregts L et al. Gastrointestinal symptoms in long-distance runners, cyclists, and triathletes: prevalence, medication, and etiology. *Am J Gastroenterol* 1999;94(6):1570–1581.

Rehrer NJ. Fluid and electrolyte balance in ultra-endurance sport. *Sports Med* 2001; 31:701–715.

Rehrer NJ, van Kemenade M, Meester W et al. Gastrointestinal complaints in relation to dietary intake in triathletes. *Int J Sport Nutr* 1992;2(1):48–59.

Shi X, Summers RW, Schedl HP, Flanagan SW, Chang R, Gisolfi CV. Effects of carbohydrate type and concentration and solution osmolality on water absorption. *Med Sci Sports Exer* 1995;27:1607–1615.

Shirreffs SM et al. Post-exercise rehydration in man: effects of volume consumed and drink sodium content. *Med Sci Sports Exerc* 1996;28:1260.

Chapter 8. Optimal Recovery

American College of Sports Medicine. Position stand on exercise and fluid replacement. *Med Sci Sport Exerc* 1996;28:i–vii.

Dunford M. Carbohydrate and Exercise. In *Sports Nutrition: A Practice Manual for Professionals*, 4th ed. Chicago: American Dietetic Association, 2006, 14–32.

———. Nutrition for Endurance Sports. In *Sports Nutrition: A Practice Manual for Professionals*, 4th ed. Chicago: American Dietetic Association, 2006, 445–459.

Hew-Butler T et al. Updated Fluid Recommendation: Position Statement from the International Marathon Medical Directors Association (IMMDA). *Clin J Sport Med* 2006; 16:283–292.

Jentjens RL et al. Addition of protein and amino acids to carbohydrate does not enhance post-exercise muscle glycogen synthesis. *J Appl Physiol* 2001;91(2):839–846.

Joint Position Statement of American College of Sports Medicine, American Dietetic Association and Dietitians of Canada. Nutrition and Athletic Performance. *Med Sci Sports Exerc* 2000; 32(12):2130–2145.

Position of the American Dietetic Association, Dietitians of Canada, and the American College of Sports Medicine: Nutrition and Athletic Performance. *JADA* 2000;100(12): 1543–1556.

Sawka MN et al. American College of Sports Medicine: Position Stand on Exercise and Fluid Replacement. *Med Sci Sports Exerc* 2007;377–390.

Tipton KD Wolfe RR. Exercise, protein metabolism, and muscle growth. *Int J Sport Nutr Exerc Metab* 2001;11:109–132.

Wildman R, Miller B. *Sports and Fitness Nutrition*. Thomson Wadsworth, 2004.

Wolinsky, I ed. *Nutrition in Exercise and Sport*, 3rd ed. Boca Raton, Fla: CRC Press, 1998.

Chapter 9. Supplements

Ahrens, JN et al. The physiological effects of caffeine in women during treadmill walking. *J Strength Condit Res* 2007;21(1):164–168.

American Dietetic Association. Position of the American Dietetic Association: Functional Foods. *J Am Diet Assoc* 2004;104:814–826.

Armstrong LE. Caffeine, body fluid-electrolyte balance, and exercise performance. *Int J Sport Nutr Exerc Metab* 2002;12:189–206.

Baylis A, Cameron-Smith D, Burke LM. Inadvertent doping through supplement use by athletes: assessment and management of the risk in Australia. *Int J Sport Nutr Exerc Metab* 2001;11:365–383.

Center for Science in the Public Interest. Caffeine Content of Food & Drugs, Sept. 2007, http://www.cspinet.org/new/cafchart.htm.

Evans GW. The effect of chromium picolinate on insulin controlled parameters in humans. *Int J Biosoc Res* 1989;11:163–180.

Graham TE. Caffeine and exercise: metabolism, endurance and performance. *Sports Med* 2001;31(11):785–807.

Haas JD, Brownlie T. Iron deficiency and reduced work capacity: a critical review of the research to determine a causal relationship. *J Nutr* 2001;131:676–690.

Hasler CM. Functional foods: their role in disease prevention and health promotion. *Food Tech* 1998;52(2):57–62.

Haymes EM, Lamanca JF. Iron loss in runners during exercise: implications and recommendations. *Sports Med* 1989;7:277–285.

Hunt JR. How important is dietary iron bioavailability? *Am J Clin Nutr* 2001;73:3–4.

Institute of Food Technologists, Expert Report. Functional Foods: Opportunities and Challenges. 2005;www.ift.org/cms/?pid=1001247. Accessed Apr. 20, 2008.

Institute of Medicine. *Dietary Reference Intakes for Calcium, Phosphorus, Magnesium, Vitamin D and Fluoride*. Washington, D.C.: National Academy Press, 1997.

———. *Dietary Reference Intakes for Thiamin, Riboflavin, Niacin, Vitamin B6, Vitamin B12,*

Pantothenic Acid, Biotin, and Choline. Washington, D.C.: National Academy Press, 1998.
———. *Dietary Reference Intakes for Vitamin C, Vitamin E, Selenium, and Carotenoids.* Washington, D.C.: National Academy Press, 2000.
———. *Dietary Reference Intakes for Vitamin A, Vitamin K, Arsenic, Boron, Chromium, Copper, Iodine, Iron, Manganese, Molybdenum, Nickel, Silicon, Vanadium, and Zinc.* Washington, D.C.: National Academy Press, 2000.
International Food Information Council (IFIC) Foundation. Background on Functional Foods. 2004; www.ific.org. Accessed Nov. 8, 2006.
———. Functional Foods Backgrounder, International Food Information Council (IFIC), Nov. 2006. http://ific.org/nutrition/functional/index.cfm. Accessed Apr. 28, 2008.
Jowko E et al. (2001) Creatine and ß-hydroxy-ß-methlbutyrate (HMB) additively increase lean body mass and muscle strength during a weight-training program. *Nutrition* 17:588–586.
Juliano LM, Griffiths RR. Caffeine. In Lowinson JH, Ruiz P, Millman RB, Langrod, JG (eds.), *Substance Abuse: A Comprehensive Textbook,* 4th ed. Baltimore: Lippincott, Williams, & Wilkins, 2005, 403–421.
LaManca JJ, Haymes EM, Daly JA et al. Sweat iron loss of male and female runners during exercise. *Int J Sports Med* 1988;9:52–55.
Machefer G, Groussard C, Vincent S et al. Multivitamin-mineral supplementation prevents lipid peroxidation during "the Marathon des Sables." *J Am Coll Nutr* 2007;26(2):111–120.
Maughan R (ed.). *Nutrition in Sport.* Blackwell, 2000.
McGuire TA et al. Creatine supplementation in high school football players. *Clin J Sports Med* 2001;11:247–253.
Millen AE et al. Use of vitamin, mineral, nonvitamin, and nonmineral supplements in the United States: the 1987, 1992, and 2000 National Health Interview Survey results. *J Am Diet Assoc* 2004;104(6):942–950.
Nutrition Business Journal. NBJ's Supplement Business Report, 2005. http://nbj.stores.yahoo .net/nbsupbusrep2.html. Accessed Apr. 29, 2008.
Office of Dietary Supplements, National Institutes of Health. http://ods.od.nih.gov/. Accessed Apr. 28, 2008.
Paddon-Jones D, et al. Potential ergogenic effects of arginine and creatine supplementation. *J Nutr* 2004;134:2888S–2894S.
Radimer K et al. Dietary supplement use by U.S. adults: data from the National Health and Nutrition Examination Survey, 1999–2000. *Am J Epidemiol* 2004;60(4):339–349.
Radimer KL et al. Nonvitamin, nonmineral dietary supplements: issues and findings from NHANES III. *J Am Diet Assoc* 2000;100(4):447–454.
Rosenbloom C, ed. *Sports Nutrition: A Guide for the Professional Working with Active People.* Chicago: American Dietetic Association, 1999.
Spriet LL. Caffeine and performance. *International Journal of Sport Nutrition* 1995;5: S84–S99.
Stellingwerff T et al. Nutritional strategies to optimize training and racing in middle-distance athletes. *J Sports Sci* 25:1:S17–S28.

Index

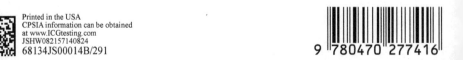